Introduction to Group Treatment for Aphasia: Design and Management

Robert C. Marshall, Ph.D.

Associate Professor, Department of Communicative Disorders,
University of Rhode Island, Kingston

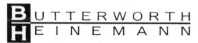
BUTTERWORTH
HEINEMANN

Boston   Oxford   Johannesburg   Melbourne   New Delhi   Singapore

Recognizing the importance of preserving what has been written,
Butterworth–Heinemann prints its books on acid-free paper whenever possible.

 Butterworth–Heinemann supports the efforts of American Forests and the Global ReLeaf Program in its campaign for the betterment of trees, forests, and our environment.

Library of Congress Cataloging-in-Publication Data
Marshall, Robert C., 1938–
        Introduction to group treatment for aphasia : design and
    management / Robert C. Marshall.
            p.   cm.
        Includes bibliographical references and index.
        ISBN 0-7506-7013-4
        1. Aphasic persons- -Rehabilitation. 2. Group speech therapy.
    I. Title
        [DNLM: 1. Aphasia- -rehabilitation. 2. Rehabilitation of Speech
    and Language Disorders- -organization & administration.
    3. Rehabilitation of Speech and Language Disorders- -methods.
    4. Speech-Language Pathology- -methods. WL 340.5 M369 1999]
    RC425.M197 1999
    616.85'5206- -dc21
    DNLM/DLC
    for Library of Congress   98-44096
                                                                    CIP

British Library Cataloguing-in-Publication Data
A catalogue record for this book is available from the British Library.

The publisher offers special discounts on bulk orders of this book.
For information, please contact:
Manager of Special Sales
Butterworth–Heinemann
225 Wildwood Avenue
Woburn, MA 01801-2041
Tel: 781-904-2500
Fax: 781-904-2620

For information on all Butterworth–Heinemann publications available,
contact our World Wide Web home page at: http://www.bh.com

10 9 8 7 6 5 4 3 2 1

Printed in the United States of America

Coventry University

Introduction to Group Treatment for Aphasia: Design and Management

To be aphasic is to possess one of life's most bewildering, encompassing, demoralizing, and frightening of human problems. Were I to become aphasic, I would no doubt also become suicidal.

—Audrey Holland, *Rationale for Adult Aphasia Therapy*, 1977

Contents

Preface

A group program for aphasic patients was started at the Department of Veterans Affairs Medical Center in Portland, Oregon, when I arrived there as a new Ph.D. in 1969. Inpatients and outpatients with aphasia, motor speech disorders, and cognitive-communicative problems resulting from traumatic brain injury and dementia and an occasional laryngectomy patient participated in this weekly group. Staff and students ran the group, which met at 10 AM every Thursday in the same place. There were few guidelines available as to what this group should be doing. No mechanisms existed to help us determine how group treatment helped the participants. Everyone involved in the process, however, thought it was a very important part of our patient care responsibilities.

A lot has happened since that first group met in 1969. Aphasia therapy has been on a roller coaster ride. In 1969, those responsible for management of persons with aphasia were shocked to learn that some physicians questioned the value of aphasia treatment. Challenged to show that aphasia treatment helped patients beyond the point of spontaneous recovery, clinical aphasiologists published group and individual studies to prove treatment efficacy in refereed journals and presented treatment efficacy data at national and international meetings. Subsequently, some of the same skeptical physicians began to sing aphasia treatment's praises. Some golden years for aphasia therapy followed. From 1975 to 1995, clinical services for patients with aphasia and related neurogenic disorders (e.g., dysarthria, dementia, dysphagia) increased markedly. Medical speech-language pathology programs flourished. Life was good.

Today, clinical aphasiologists are once more hearing those questioning voices. The message is that health care, of which aphasia treatment is a part, costs too much. Those who provide speech-language pathology services are asked again to prove their worth by showing that aphasia treatment is cost-effective and to reduce the cost of services by seeing more patients, limiting services for some patients, and reducing treatment charges.

Group treatment, once a popular means of treating patients with aphasia, gave way to individual treatment from 1975 to 1995. Present-day practice suggests there is renewed interest in group work. New books on group treatment are available; convention program offerings on the subject are abundant. One of the principal objectives of this book is to present group treatment as a viable, cost-effective alternative to individual treatment and as a treatment of choice for some patients with aphasia. Readers of this book should understand, however, that the initiation of a group program should not be undertaken lightly and that a significant amount of work should be done before a group meets for the first time.

Much of the material in this book comes from my 28 years of experience in facilitating and cofacilitating group treatment programs for patients with neurogenic communication disorders at the Department of Veterans Affairs Medical Center in Portland, Oregon, and at the University of Rhode Island. What I learned about group therapy came from (1) realistically appraising the successes and failures of the programs I was associated with; (2) listening to both positive and negative comments on group treatment from patients, family members, and colleagues; and (3) sharing and exchanging ideas about group treatment with colleagues who were overseeing groups in clinical work settings.

Throughout my work with a variety of groups for persons with aphasia and related disorders, I had a lot of ideas about what I could do to make group treatment sessions more effective and accountable. Many of these ideas were simple adjustments in procedure that would make the group meetings run more smoothly. For example, it is useful to have some guidelines for canceling a group meeting in case of bad weather. Some group seating arrangements seem to work better than others. Certain group compositions of aphasic patients do very well in a group situation; others should be avoided entirely. I certainly did not act on all the ideas I thought had merit, but in this book I share the things that worked, some that failed, and untested ideas that, I believe, still have some merit. Throughout the book, to bridge the gap between theory and practice, I have provided relevant examples of specific patients involved in my groups.

This book is aimed at professionals responsible for management of patients with aphasia and other cognitive-communicative disorders caused by brain damage. Speech-language pathologists responsible for management of persons with aphasia and related disorders will be the paramount users of this book. However, the material in the book can be put to good use by clinicians and clinician-managers from other disciplines (i.e., occupational therapy, recreational therapy, psychology) as well. Group treatment is given little consideration in courses on aphasia. Given the present state of affairs, it is time to change this. It is my hope, therefore, that this book will help foster this change in attitudes toward and practices of group treatment and that students in training are exposed to this text.

R.C.M.

Acknowledgments

Many things have influenced my thoughts about group treatment in the last 28 years. I am fortunate to have worked most of those years for the Department of Veterans Affairs Health Care System, where treatment groups of all kinds were supported and encouraged. I am equally fortunate to be involved with group programs outside my university employment setting where long-term support for patients with aphasia and their families is valued and appreciated.

I have certainly learned a great deal from the patients seen in group situations. Space does not allow me to cite all the individuals who stimulated my interest in group treatment programs at the Portland Veterans Affairs Medical Center (PVAMC) and at the University of Rhode Island (URI). However, I will always remember and appreciate the contributions of John D., George J., Ben H., Bob J., Robert C., Cecile M., Ed B., Norm R., Mike B., Dick B., Tom M., Pat N., Gerry B., Jeri B., Gerald B., Ralph W., Bill W., Jim M., and Hal B. All of the patients and family members who participated in aphasia and other groups at PVAMC and who participate at URI have my heartfelt appreciation and lasting respect. Thank you for your patience and understanding and for teaching me so much.

I want to express my gratitude to present and former members of the speech-language pathology staff of PVAMC, specifically Sandra Neuburger, Lynn Fox, Judy Rau, Lee Ann Golper, and Kathy Frazier, for sharing insights on their own group programs, for filling in for me when I was absent, and for helping to keep me clinically connected for more than a quarter of a century. Special kudos are also in order to the scores of speech-language pathology trainees in PVAMC program who took their turn in running our groups. What they shared, wrote, and accomplished is a part of this book. I am also indebted to Muriel Lezak and Diane Howieson, two special neuropsychologists with whom I was privileged to cofacilitate group treatment programs for many years. No less valuable are those colleagues who shared their insights and experiences in group treatment with me at many clinical aphasiology conferences.

Much of the material on which this book is based has been published since 1995. In the late 1980s, the journal *Aphasiology*, published by Taylor and Frances, was launched. This journal's clinical forum issues, broad-based spectrum of papers on aphasia, and special feature editions have contributed immeasurably to the writing of this book. *Aphasiology* has been a continuous source of information for persons interested in the study of individuals with aphasia.

The single-handed writing of any book is a labor-intensive endeavor. I could not have devoted the time to this task were it not for the hard work and continuous support of my research staff at URI. Kristin King-Iden and Claudia A. Morelli kept the Aphasia Research Lab in order so that I had the time to write this book. I am also indebted to my wife, Micah, for sparing me from all responsibilities save those associated with my profession. She has definitely been the secret weapon who allowed this book to be finished in a timely fashion. Finally, I would also like to thank Barbara Murphy, former senior editor, and Leslie Kramer, assistant editor, both of Butterworth–Heinemann, for initiating this project and for their encouragement during the writing of the book.

R.C.M.

1

Introduction

The disabilities and handicaps associated with aphasia and its related adult neurogenic communication disorders are permanent. Rehabilitation minimizes but does not "cure" these deficits. Most persons with aphasia face a lifetime of adjusting to and compensating for cognitive-communicative, physical, and psychosocial problems brought about by aphasia and stroke. Lyon articulated this point very well in viewing the consequences of aphasia in terms of a long journey shared by both patient and caregiver.[1] Rehabilitation specialists understand clearly the long-term consequences of these problems and recognize brain-injured persons' need for ongoing professional support.[2-4] Group treatment is a cost-effective, efficient means of providing this support in the early postonset period and particularly after the aphasia is chronic.[5-6] In conversations and communications about group treatment with rehabilitation specialists, I have found that clinician-managers want a group treatment program to which they can refer patients after discharge from individual treatment. Some have expressed a need to start their own groups.[2, 6-8] Rarely are such programs available.

PURPOSE AND SCOPE

Our capacity to speak and to communicate distinguishes us from other species. Besides breathing, communication is the most frequently repeated action of all human beings.[9] Connecting with others through communication is important for us; it is how we explore our world and express our self-hood.[10] Aphasia affects these capacities. Aphasia groups provide an important channel for "reconnecting" the patient with what was, what is, and what can be. This book highlights the roles of two players in the group treatment process. The first is the patient with aphasia. I use the term *patient* not because it is the best term, but because it is familiar to me.

The second group of persons to whom this book is directed is those who organize and provide treatment for persons with aphasia. I use the term *clinician-manager* to refer to health care professionals (e.g., physician; speech-language pathologist; occupational, physical, and recreational therapist; social worker) who have clinical service, managerial, or other decision-making responsibilities affecting clinical outcomes for brain-injured persons. The term *clinician* refers to the person conducting group therapy sessions.

In today's health care climate, health care organization administrators appear to have a different mind-set than that of most clinicians and clinician-managers.[8] Faced with the realities of dwindling resources, those concerned with the quality of patient care appear to be "at war" with insurance companies, health maintenance organizations (HMOs), and other payers over many issues. One point of contention is the initiation of new service programs such as group therapy. If you are a clinician or clinician-manager who thinks that group treatment is a cost-effective and viable means of treating some aphasic patients in your work setting, this book will supply some "ammunition" with which to wage your war.

Some of the reluctance in starting group treatment programs stems from the fact that few individuals are truly aware of the factors that must be considered and problems that should be solved before starting any type of group treatment program. The myriad of decisions required in developing and starting a group may overwhelm the best of intentions. Limited information is available to guide clinician-managers in terms of what to do. Accounts of group treatment tend to focus on the therapeutic activities of the group rather than on what is involved in starting a group. Furthermore, the information in these clinically focused reports is too often only applicable to a particular group, not the process and conduct of group treatment in general. A basic premise of this book is that clinician-managers who wish to have a group treatment program in their work setting will need to do a significant amount of work before approaching higher-level administration about sponsoring a group treatment program.[11] Without doing this work, presenting group treatment as a cost-effective method of treating patients with acquired neurogenic communication disorders will be difficult.

The overall goal of this book is to elevate the status of group treatment in the aphasic clinician's arsenal of accountable treatments. Its specific objectives are (1) to guide clinician-managers through the prerequisite planning, negotiating, and problem solving to start a successful, sustaining, and cost-effective group program; (2) to provide a comprehensive review of group treatment and specific group treatment activities that can be used by practicing clinicians; and (3) to offer options for clinicians to document the effects of group treatment by using objective communicative and psychosocial measures and by collecting social validation data.

Material presented in this textbook is applicable to group treatment for adults with aphasia and other acquired neurogenic communication disorders. The latter include motor speech disorders (apraxia of speech and dysarthria), and cognitive-communicative disorders secondary to diffuse neurologic involvement (e.g., dementing conditions and traumatic brain injury). Some suggestions may also be applicable to starting other adult group treatments (e.g., stuttering and laryngectomized persons).

Group treatment, as discussed in this book, is intended for patients with more chronic neurogenic communication problems. *Chronic* means that the patient is (1) at least 3 months postonset; (2) finished with his or her individual treatment; and (3) cognizant of the fact that he or she will need to live with, adjust to, and compensate for long-term speech and language deficits. This definition does not mean that group therapy is inappropriate for patients who are less than 3 months postonset. Some of these patients are sufficiently aware of their deficits and are motivated to be able to participate in groups. Inclusion of these types of patients is, however, beyond the scope of this book.

Group therapy, as discussed in this book, is further restricted to groups that have, at least in part, as their purposes the following: (1) improving communication, (2) increasing participation in life, and (3) reducing psychosocial consequences of stroke and associated disorders such as aphasia. Most forms of group therapy discussed herein should therefore be considered reimbursable, as alternatives to individual treatment for some patients, and as preferred methods of treatment for others.

Material on group treatment for this book primarily reflects literature since the 1970s. For more inclusive reviews of group treatment, particularly earlier reports, the reader should consult other sources.[12-14]

This book can be used by clinicians and clinician-managers in planning, organizing, initiating, and running group treatment programs in a variety of work settings: rehabilitation centers, university clinics, hospitals, outpatient and community clinics, community agencies, and nursing homes. It can also be used in the training of students and professionals in health-related fields interested in starting group treatment programs.

ORGANIZATION

The book is organized into three major sections. Section I (Chapters 2–5) is devoted to the planning and organization of group treatment programs. Chapter 2 addresses the benefits of group treatment for the patient with aphasia, the health care organization (e.g., hospital) and its component programs (e.g., rehabilitation unit). Chapter 3 focuses on logistics: recruitment, transportation, space, equipment, and scheduling. Chapter 4 deals with the major concern of health care professionals today—funding. Chapter 5 provides information on group composition, behavioral expectations, and leadership.

Section II (Chapters 6–8) is devoted to an examination of group treatment methods and programs. Chapter 6 overviews some of the expectations of group treatment and presents guidelines for obtaining prerequisite background data on patients starting in a group. Chapter 7 provides a synopsis of communicative, psychosocial, and transitional group programs. Chapter 8 provides more specific information on treatment methods that appear particularly well suited for use in group situations.

Section III (Chapters 9–11) focuses on documentation. The initial chapter in this section (Chapter 9) gives the clinician strategies for documenting the events of specific group treatment sessions. Chapter 10 offers a large array of strategies for documenting group treatment outcomes on a monthly basis. The monthly documentation strategies are presented in four subsections: test-retest, verbal measures, communication measures, and psychosocial measures. Chapter 11 describes methods for obtaining social validation of the benefits of group treatment.

Chapter 12 presents a futuristic look at group treatment. It summarizes my fears and hopes for the future of this worthy endeavor.

REFERENCES

1. Lyon J. Coping with Aphasia. San Diego: Singular, 1998;1.
2. Marshall RC. Problem-Solving Support Groups for Long-Term Brain Injured Adults. Paper presented at the American Speech-Language-Hearing Association Convention, Boston, November 1997.
3. Beeson P, Holland AL. Aphasia Groups: An Approach to Long-Term Rehabilitation. Telerounds #19. Tucson, AZ: National Center for Neurogenic Communication Disorders, 1994.
4. Wehman P, Kreutzer J, Wood W, et al. Helping traumatically brain injured patients return to work with supported employment: three case studies. Arch Phys Med Rehabil 1989;70:109.
5. Simmons-Mackie N. A solution to the discharge dilemma in aphasia: social approaches to aphasia management. Aphasiology 1998;12:231.
6. Marshall RC. Problem-focused group therapy for mildly aphasic clients. Am J Speech-Lang Pathol 1993;2:31.
7. Marshall RC. Treatment of Aphasia: A Long-Term Problem Solving Perspective. Paper presented at the Canadian Speech-Language-Hearing Association Convention, Ottawa, March 1995.

8. Marshall RC. An introduction to supported conversation for adults with aphasia: perspectives, problems and possibilities. Aphasiology 1998;12:812.
9. Lynch JJ. The Language of the Heart. New York: Basic Books, 1985;118.
10. Lindfors JW. Speaking Creatures in the Classroom. In S Hynd, DL Rubin (eds), Perspectives on Talk and Learning. Urbana, IL: National Council of Teachers of English, 1992;21.
11. Hartford ME. Groups in human services: some facts and fancies. Soc Work Groups 1978;1:7.
12. Kearns K. Group Therapy for Aphasia: Theoretical and Practical Considerations. In R Chapey (ed), Language Intervention Strategies in Adult Aphasia (3rd ed). Baltimore: Williams & Wilkins, 1993;304.
13. Fawcus M. Group Therapy: A Learning Situation. In C Code, D Muller (eds), Aphasia Therapy (2nd ed). London: Whurr, 1989;113.
14. Pachalska M. Group therapy for aphasia patients. Aphasiology 1991;5:541.

I

Planning and Organization

2

Benefits of Group Treatment

Group therapy for clients with aphasia and related neurogenic communicative disorders is not a new concept. Group programs became a necessity in the 1940s when few trained clinicians were available to treat the head-injured servicemen returning from World War II.[1–2] Interest in group work abated in favor of individual therapy from the 1950s to the 1980s. Importantly, this lack of interest occurred in conjunction with an influx of Medicare dollars that paid for individual treatment and a 1983 decision by Congress not to apply a diagnosis-related group–based prospective payment system (PPS) to rehabilitation services.[3] Current treatment practices suggest a heightened interest in the use of group treatment for patients with aphasia and related neurogenic communication disorders.[4–7] This resurgence of group therapy can be attributed to two factors: (1) reimbursement and time management issues associated with health care costs, and (2) evidence that group treatment might be equally as effective or perhaps more effective for certain patients with aphasia.

This chapter highlights some of the benefits of group treatment. It begins with a brief review of the general value of group treatment per se. Some, but certainly not all, information in this review is applicable to aphasia group treatment. This review is followed by a summary of some of the empirical and clinical evidence that shows that group treatment can (1) improve communicative abilities of persons with aphasia, and (2) benefit the patient from a psychosocial standpoint and facilitate his or her reintegration into society. A third segment of the chapter identifies potential benefits, specifically cost and time savings, for health care organizations and their component programs (e.g., rehabilitation units) that support group programs. The final section of the chapter illustrates how group programs interface with or relate to other patient care programs within health care organizations (e.g., patient and family education, follow-up medical care, research, and student training), and it addresses potential cost and time savings that result from these relationships.

GENERAL BENEFITS OF GROUP TREATMENT

Therapy groups in communication disorders attempt to ameliorate specific speech and language problems; other groups serve counseling and other functions. Most groups, however, are multipurpose.[8] Groups are widely used within and outside the field of communication disorders, particularly in the field of psychotherapy.[9–11] The general benefits of group treatment are multifaceted.[11]

Hope

When patients enter an existing group, they find that someone with a similar problem has overcome a certain amount of adversity. This knowledge may lift a patient's spirits and cause him or her to realize that positive changes can occur regardless of one's circumstances.

Universality

Groups help individuals realize they are not alone in the experience of stroke, traumatic brain injury, progressive disease, and the accompanying residuals of these neurologic sequelae. Knowing that he or she is not alone can be a relief and a source of comfort for a patient and his or her family.

Altruism

Altruism is thought of as unselfishly providing a service to another human being. The opportunity to be useful to others, specifically to engage in altruistic behavior, can be an important source of renewed self-esteem. By imparting and sharing information, group participants help one another. Most clinician-managers see the desire to help in patients who have suffered strokes, head injuries, or undergone a laryngectomy, and who attempt to start their own groups to help others with similar problems. Harnessing this energy in a group facilitated by a professional may pay substantial dividends.

Imparting Information

In a group, information can be provided by the leader or outside speaker. A group is a vehicle for providing helpful didactic instruction to all group members. Group members also provide information to other group members by directing them to resources, sharing past experiences, and offering helpful advice. Group participants, and certainly group facilitators, always leave group meetings more informed than they were when the meeting started.

Socialization Skills

Some patients with aphasia communicate readily in one-to-one situations with the support and guidance of the therapist, but they avoid communicating in social situations involving friends, family, and other naturalistic environments. Risk of embarrassment, lack of trust, and fear limit some aphasic people from using the compensatory skills taught in treatment in social situations. In fact, severely aphasic patients selectively choose where and with whom they will use compensatory communication strategies.[12] Group situations provide an opportunity for participants to learn and use interpersonal skills in a safe environment and enhance the transfer of these skills into other areas of life.

Venting Feelings

Many aphasic stroke patients harbor unspoken feelings and fears of many sorts. Nonaphasic communicators have limited time to listen to the expression of these feelings and fears. A group provides a safe and supportive environment to release these feelings with persons likely to listen and to understand.

> Mr. N., a 44-year-old man with improving Wernicke's aphasia, was a single parent of an 11-year-old boy. His son, through a joint custody agreement, spent a portion of the week with Mr. N. and a portion of it with Mr. N.'s ex-wife. After the stroke, the ex-wife filed for sole custody of the boy, citing Mr. N.'s stroke as proof that sole custody was the proper course of action. Arguments raged between Mr. N.'s relatives and the ex-wife and respective lawyers for both parties over what to do. Mr. N., ignored in these arguments, was seething. In the safety of the group, he screamed, "Everyone's feelings are being considered except mine!" Mr. N. needed a safe place to express his feelings where he would be given the time to do so and those listening would understand.

Although the emotional release or catharsis achieved from expressing a feeling is not a cure, it promotes growth. Once Mr. N. had expressed his feelings on how his son's custody situation was being handled and the family's lack of consideration, he took action. With minimal assistance from his therapist, he re-established the prior joint custody arrangement with his ex-wife.

Cohesiveness

Cohesiveness relates to the attractiveness of the group to its members. Cohesiveness is analogous to trust in individual therapy.[10] Groups who are cohesive work together. Similar to a basketball team that begins as a group of separate individuals with different skills, groups develop "chemistry" and become a working unit. When one member faces a difficult problem and succeeds in solving it with the help of the group, it has a positive impact on other group members. This success increases group cohesiveness.

> Mr. C., a 64-year-old man with mild aphasia, was a widower of some 3 years' duration. A handsome man, Mr. C. wanted companionship, but he had no idea about how to start dating again. Within his group, this problem was examined. Suggestions as to how Mr. C. might meet "Ms. Right" were discussed. Eventually, Mr. C. took the risk of writing a personal ad for the newspaper. The communicative interactions, goodwill, and mutual growth of the group as Mr. C. responded to those who answered the ad and how he dealt with explaining that he had had a stroke to potential dates were stimulating to all.

Mr. C. eventually met and married a respondent to his ad. Two other group members, also widowers, eventually remarried. The increase in group cohesiveness as a result of this single episode was enormous. Leuterman, a consummate group therapist and counselor, states that he knows a group is cohesive when he "can hardly wait for the session to start and [he] look[s] forward to seeing the other members of the group."[8] This anticipation was indeed the case when I thought about seeing Mr. C. and his group.

INDIVIDUAL BENEFITS

Many writers point out that group therapy should not be a replacement for individual treatment.[13-16] However, this point of view may put group treatment in a negative light. It is seen only as a supplement to individual treatment and an opportunity for socialization for persons with aphasia. Many have argued that the efficacy of group treatment has limited scientific support.[2, 17-19] Evidence is available, however, that suggests that the communicative and psychosocial functioning of patients with aphasia does improve as a consequence of group treatment. Some of this evidence is reviewed here. Additional information is provided in Chapter 7.

Communication Benefits

In 1981, a multicenter Veterans Administration cooperative study[20] compared the effects of group and individual treatment with aphasic patients. Subjects were randomly assigned to group or individual treatment. Subjects began treatment at 4 weeks postonset. Each subject received 8 hours of group or individual speech and language treatment per week for 44 weeks. Subjects were evaluated at 15, 26, 37, and 48 weeks postonset with a battery of speech, language, and other tests. Results showed that group treatment resulted in gains in speech and language functions on standardized tests equivalent to those gained in individual treatment. This landmark study is discussed in more detail later.

One investigation of group treatment randomly assigned patients with aphasia to group treatment or to a deferred treatment cohort that served as a control group.[21] Results showed that subjects who had group treatment for their language deficits made significantly greater improvement on a battery of standardized speech and language measures than that seen in deferred treatment subjects. When the deferred group subjects had received group treatment for an equivalent length of time, their test results showed that they made progress equivalent to that of the treated group. Avent used a multiple baseline single-subject design to examine the effects of cooperative group treatment on the narrative skills of eight aphasic subjects.[22] She found that cooperative group treatment significantly improved the content of subjects' narrative and procedural discourse. This improvement also extended to other situations. Other studies of group therapy not using comparative, deferred or control groups, or single-subject design methods, have also shown that patients with aphasia improve on both standardized and functional speech and language tests as a consequence of group therapy.[23-26]

One survey of speech-language pathologists specializing in the treatment of neurogenic communication disorders indicated that most respondents believed communication improved most with a combination of group and individual treatment.[27] Finally, comments from aphasic patients who have been participants in group treatment programs and their family members highlight the value of group treatment participation.[2, 28-30] Although these anecdotal comments cannot be taken as proof of the efficacy of group treatment, such positive statements are difficult to ignore in view of marketplace emphasis on consumer satisfaction.[31]

Psychosocial Benefits

The psychosocial benefits of group treatment are numerous and varied. Several writers have stressed the need to increase communication opportunities for patients with neurogenic communication disorders.[32-33] For expressively restricted aphasic adults who have few communication partners, a weekly group treatment session constitutes an important, and perhaps the only, opportunity for the patient to use intact social communication skills (e.g., greetings and appropriate use of yes and no). For some brain-injured patients, the group encounters are the only time when the individual receives the necessary support to convey his or her important thoughts and ideas. Noteworthy examples are group treatment programs at the York-Durham Aphasia Center, North York, Ontario, Canada.[34–35] Here, group facilitators are schooled in the use of an intervention called *supportive conversation for aphasic adults* (SCA). Aura Kagan, the developer of SCA, suggests that the skilled facilitator becomes a "communicative ramp" for the aphasic members of the group. Through the use of the communicative ramp, aphasic patients can access thoughts and feelings that are masked by aphasia.[36]

Some clinicians have suggested that therapists work harder to make the communicative interactions within the treatment session similar to those occurring in the natural environment.[37] Group work offers a variety of communicative and social interactions for its participants that are not available in individual treatment. For example, the group situation allows the patient to exchange information with multiple partners who have different backgrounds and interests. It enhances the patient's use of pragmatic skills: taking turns, listening closely, making eye contact, switching topics, and maintaining a topic. Within a group the patient is able to exchange ideas, barter, argue, debate, and compete. Such speech acts are rarely a part of individual treatment sessions, in which the therapist tends to dominate. The group situation allows its members to use and practice compensatory and adaptive communication strategies in a situation in which they can receive feedback about the effectiveness of these strategies from many sources rather than from a single therapist. Group therapy can also be used to enhance collaborative problem solving, especially with higher level aphasic patients.[23, 29] All aforementioned communicative acts are further enhanced by the bonding that occurs among group members both inside and outside the group.

Protracted individual therapy may cause some patients to become overly dependent on the therapist. This dependency can lessen the transfer of skills learned in treatment to outside situations.[38] A patient who becomes a part of a group and learns to solve problems collaboratively and to seek assistance from knowledgeable colleagues in the group may become more independent.[39] Group therapy may positively affect psychosocial reintegration by supplying a supportive environment in which use of compensatory communicative options are encouraged and modeled by the clinician and participating group members. For example, one study illustrated that patients with aphasia who attended group treatment once per month over a 30-month time span illustrated marked improvement in pre- and post-treatment depression and anxiety measures.[40] These improvements were accompanied by increased social activity and independence. Furthermore, group situations allow clients with neurogenic communication disorders to see that others have similar problems.[41] They can observe how others cope with disability, lessening the feelings of isolation brought about by the trauma of stroke and head injury. For some clients, a stint in group treatment may provide the needed transition from individual treatment to termination of treatment.

HEALTH CARE ORGANIZATION BENEFITS

Americans are concerned about the rising cost of health care.[42] The cost of speech and language therapy is included among these concerns.[43–45] Health care organizations aspire to deliver the best patient care at the lowest costs. Sometimes the value of patient care is measured according to its impact on the life of the individual receiving it and according to its ultimate cost to society. For example, a cognitive therapy program that succeeded in restoring a 24-year-old head-injured patient to gainful employment and removing him from the long-term disability roles would be considered valuable for two reasons. First, it would save money for the organization over the working life of the client. Second, it would improve the individual's self-esteem, and improved self-esteem goes hand-in-hand with greater independence. This independence might be expressed in increased activity, better relations with others, and in other ways.

Reducing Costs of Treatment

The cost of individual speech and language treatment varies widely across the United States. In 1995, individual speech and language treatment was being reimbursed at $165 per hour by the Portland Veterans Administration Medical Center (PVAMC) when an eligible veteran could not obtain speech and language treatment at the medical center. If this $165 charge was distributed across a group of four patients, the cost per patient would be slightly more than $41. Group treatment, if billed at rates equivalent to individual treatment, is less costly than individual treatment. This billing method would result in a savings of nearly 300%.

Extending Treatment

A PPS is likely to be implemented to reduce the cost of medical care associated with outpatient rehabilitation.[3] Under a PPS, the rehabilitation program would receive a predetermined number of dollars to cover rehabilitation services associated with a medical diagnosis such as stroke. For example, $1,600 or 10 therapy sessions might be given to cover speech and language therapy for an aphasic stroke patient. Using the previously stated $165 per hour as an individual treatment rate, these funds would cover less than 10 individual sessions. The same funds, however, would cover 38 group treatments. A PPS should prompt for-ward-looking clinician-managers to consider stretching treatment dol-lars by placing appropriate patients in long-term, less intensive group treatment instead of short-term, intensive individual treatment.

> Mr. W. was a 66-year-old man with mild anomic aphasia and no physical deficits after a left hemisphere cerebrovascular accident (CVA). His physician recommended that he seek disability retire-ment. Mr. W., however, was 3 years short of receiving a modest retirement pension and would be penalized monetarily by going on disability. The "mildness" of Mr. W.'s deficits did not warrant further individual work, but he was apprehensive about returning to work with no ongoing support. In a group situation, Mr. W. learned that he did, in fact, retain those skills necessary to continue his work as a file clerk. Group members and the therapist were able to suggest a number of strategies to facilitate Mr. W.'s gradual tran-sition back to work. Mr. W., with the support of the group, moved from working part-time to full-time. His employers were so pleased to have him back that they allowed him to attend group sessions weekly with pay.

Using all of Mr. W.'s treatment dollars for individual treatment might have deprived him of the therapeutic support needed to phase back into full-time work. In the group, Mr. W. learned from patients who had been in similar situations. Group treatment met an important need for this patient.

Another situation in which the clinician-manager might consider spending her or his treatment dollars for group treatment in lieu of individual treatment is when long-term improvement is anticipated for the patient. Here, the astute clinician-manager realizes that funds for individual treatment will be exhausted before the patient has improved maximally.[46–47] Group treatment would help stretch the funds and pro-vide services for the patient over a greater portion of the improvement course. Consider the following example:

> Mr. V., a 47-year-old man, experienced a massive left hemisphere CVA, leaving him with global aphasia and severe apraxia of speech. His funds for individual treatment were soon exhausted, and his impairments remained significant. Mr. V. had little family support and was placed in a nursing home. He fought desperately to remove himself from the nursing home with no success. His solu-

tion was creative. He became romantically involved with an aide who worked at the nursing home and persuaded her to remove him from the facility. Soon after he left the facility, Mr. V. terminated the relationship and was again on his own.

All the individual treatment in the world will not make Mr. V.'s global aphasia go away. Yet Mr. V., with his extremely limited communication skills, proved that he could indeed live somewhere other than a nursing home. With a little support from a group for Mr. V., the payer might have saved the money spent for a nursing home. Moreover, Mr. V. would not have had to experience the negative experiences of the situation. Aphasic patients such as Mr. V. might, with the support of a group, live more independently and at less cost to society. The potential savings for such patients are enormous over a life span.

Improved Customer Relations

Medical care is a business.[48] Just as companies make profits for their stockholders by having a large base of customers, health care organizations profit when individuals choose them as a medical care provider. Marketing, public relations, and community goodwill influence consumer choices. Group programs can connect patients (customers) to the sponsoring health care organization. Of course, health care organizations would rather attract healthy patients than sick ones as subscribers. Aphasic stroke patients, once stabilized, are not sick. When given the support of a group, they may become motivated to once again participate in life's events and live many years in good health. Similarly, head-injured patients are typically young and live many years in good health after a brain trauma. The sponsorship of a group program by the same health care organization that provides a patient's medical care increases the likelihood that the patient will remain a customer of that organization. This goodwill may be returned, in part, by the patient's and his or her family's recommending the health care organizations' programs and services to others.

Businesses do not like to lose customers. A patient dismissed from individual treatment by one health care group may seek treatment from another. Consider the following possible scenario:

> John B. has aphasia. His health maintenance organization covers 24 speech-language treatments per calendar year. John B. received his initial 24 treatments at the Paul Broca Medical Center (PBMC), but the PBMC does not have a group treatment program. The Carl Wernicke Medical Center (CWMC), just across town, has a group program. John B. and his family think that he can still make progress. He enrolls in the group program at CWMC. What are the

possibilities (1) that John B. and his family will be lost as customers to PBMC, and (2) that the CWMC will capture the revenues for John B.'s speech and language treatment in the new year?

Alternatively, think of the possible benefits to the PBMC if it had a group treatment program in which to transition John B. instead of dismissing him. First, the group provides a means to monitor John B.'s progress to determine whether more individual treatment is needed. If additional individual treatment is not needed, the group will aid his transition from individual treatment to dismissal. Second, group treatment at PBMC keeps John B. from "therapy shopping." If and when he actually needs more individual treatment that will be funded in the new year, PBMC will capture the funds. Third, if re-evaluation at PBMC mitigates against more individual treatment, the decision will be based on his performance data, which are not readily available to the staff at CWMC. Fourth, this decision will be made by clinicians who have followed John B. from the onset of his stroke. These are examples of the types of informed decisions that can only save money for the parties involved.

Improved Resource Use

In some situations, a patient could actually receive more intensive treatment in a group than in an individual situation. If a health care organization has a shortage of available therapists, group work could save therapist time spent on individual treatment.[49] For example, a patient who could only be seen for 1 hour each week individually could be seen three times per week in a group of three persons. This plan triples the amount of treatment time for the patient and affords him or her more practice opportunities. The therapist spends the same amount of time, 3 hours, treating the same number of patients. Of course, this situation may not always be advantageous. In some cases, however, the distributed practice, increased opportunities for socialization, and shared problem solving, as well as direct therapist-patient contact, may be more beneficial than a once-a-week individual session.

SAVING TIME FOR STAFF

Another business axiom is that "time is money." Health care organizations that sponsor group treatment programs give participants in those programs a central point for obtaining information about medical care, health, and other concerns. Consider how a group might save time for workers in the health care organization.

Reducing Medical Care Inquiries

Patients who have had strokes or traumatic head injuries, or who have a progressive neurologic disease such as Parkinson's frequently have limited knowledge of their medical conditions. After discharge from the hospital, a patient or family members will call the hospital emergency room, switchboard, nurse, admitting office, or the physician with questions regarding posthospital issues. These calls may reflect concerns related to activity (e.g., "Can I exercise?"), physical sensations (e.g., hypostasis), or medical news flashes in the newspaper or aired on television (e.g., An aspirin a day prevents stroke.). The hours spent by professionals, paraprofessionals, and clerical staff answering and returning telephone calls and leaving and answering voice messages add up. Failure to respond to these inquiries has a negative effect on customer relationships. Many of these routine questions can be answered in group treatment sessions. In fact, some make great discussion topics for the group. If necessary, the patient can be referred to the appropriate source to answer his or her question by the group leader.

> Ms. M., a 71-year-old woman with moderate fluent aphasia, lived alone. She had no close friends or relatives to rely on. Her closest contacts were the personnel working at the hospital. These people were her prime source of stimulation. Ms. M., somewhat aggressive by nature, always sought immediate answers to medical questions. She called the hospital switchboard several times per week for problems such as cellulitis, dizziness, and use of medications. Her aphasic deficits prevented an expeditious routing of her calls to the triage nurse or physician. Her descriptions of her complaints were not always accurate. Before starting group treatment, Ms. M. called the medical center approximately four times per week. Staff spent an estimated 2 hours per week with Ms. M. explaining her symptoms, returning telephone calls, and scheduling appointments, often not needed, in appropriate clinics.

When Ms. M. was put into group therapy, the routine calls to the hospital switchboard stopped. Many of her questions could be answered in the group. When Ms. M. had a question that represented a legitimate concern, the therapist was able to make a call for her or to ask a hospital staff member directly.

Patient Education

Patient education is an important part of medical care. Aphasic stroke patients receive counseling regarding diet, hypertension, use of medications, and habitual behaviors (e.g., alcohol use). Providing this information to a patient with a neurogenic communication disorder can require extra time. Those not trained in the nuances of communicating with aphasic people may be unsure of whether the information has been effectively transmitted. A group therapy session provides an excellent place to carry on these types of educational activities for patients with communication disorders. Here, the dietitian or nurse reaches more than one patient at a time. The speech-language pathologist is there to give assistance and resolve communication breakdowns. Group members who have already heard about things such as low-fat diets reap the rewards of hearing this information a second time. Sharing experiences and frustrations and learning how others deal with changes in living brought about by stroke enhance learning and may improve patient compliance with instructions. Moreover, the communicative value of these sessions should not be underestimated because it allows group members to communicate about something important to them. Combining patient education with a group speech and language session again serves a dual function and constitutes a time savings.

In-Services

In-services are an integral part of the medical education process, especially in long-term care and subacute facilities.[50–51] These programs target service staff (e.g., nursing assistants) who provide personal care to patients. Goals of in-service programs are to improve staff problem solving, to help staff develop skills needed to manage communication breakdowns, and to change staff attitudes toward communicatively impaired persons.[51] Sometimes a therapist will ask a staff member to accompany her or him to a patient's room to watch a demonstration of a particular technique. If the patient is unavailable (e.g., asleep, in the bathroom, or engaged in another activity), this time is wasted. Using a portion of a group treatment session to provide in-service education to the staff eliminates this problem and provides other advantages that translate to time saved. First, multiple staff members can be involved. Within the group, staff can observe more than one patient in a more relaxed atmosphere. An interactive educational experience may be more conducive to learning how to communicate with aphasic patients than a lecture situation.

Facilitating Follow-Up Care

Brain-injured patients require medical follow-up in clinics (e.g., neurology, hypertension, and general medicine). Follow-up visits are briefer than the 60- to 90-minute slots scheduled for group speech-language pathology treatment. The "piggy-backing" of medical appointments with group speech-language pathology appointments is another way to save the time of support personnel and medical staff, as well as of patients and family members. This approach also reduces the cost of transportation for the client and his or her family.

Clerical Support

Few hospital speech-language pathology units have assigned clerical support. Nevertheless, a certain amount of "busy work" is inherent in all clinical activities. If the clinician spends time photocopying, preparing treatment materials, retrieving charts, and transporting patients to and from therapy, the amount of time available for providing direct services is reduced. Because treatment is billable and clerical activities performed by the clinician are not, asking a volunteer to perform these types of activities may be advantageous. Putting a responsible, mildly aphasic group member on scholarship and having him or her perform these tasks in lieu of paying for the therapy provides another opportunity for savings. Many high-level patients would gladly perform a few hours of volunteer labor in exchange for a waiver of group treatment fees. For example, aphasic patients at the North York Aphasia Center serve as telephone operators. One of the group members in the program at the PVAMC helped with filing duties. Chronic aphasic people are often willing to do something to help out. This constructive activity promotes feelings of self-worth for the patient.

Benefits in Counseling, Training, and Research

Speech-language pathologists are aware of the need to involve family members in treatment. How often does the clinician or clinician-manager need to call the patient's spouse or family member to suggest something to enhance the patient's communication? Telephone calls take time. Sometimes no one is home. You leave a message. Your call is returned, and you are with a patient. The result is "telephone tag."

I have found that in many of our group programs the patient's significant other (SO) accompanied the patient to the group session. I could speak to the SO about ongoing communication and other issues on the spot. The SO also had an opportunity to ask me questions. In addition, the SOs (usually spouses of the patients in the group) created an unstructured "minigroup" of their own in the waiting room. They provided mutual support for each other by discussing problems, concerns, and solutions. Availability of family members at group treatment sessions gives the clinician ready-made opportunities to involve them in the treatment process. It saves time because it obviates the need to call or schedule a separate conference for a family member, and it enhances on-the-spot clinical teaching.

Many clinicians participate in the training of students. I believe that without the goodwill and nonremunerated efforts of these dedicated individuals, the field of speech-language pathology would suffer. Group programs, in the form of social language groups and periodic follow-up of patients dismissed from individual treatment, are a good place to introduce students in training to the problems and behaviors of clients with neurogenic communicative disorders.[51-53] The group provides a more relaxed atmosphere in which to introduce beginning students to the management of patients with acquired neurogenic communication disorders.

Clinical research benefits from the existence of group treatment programs. When a clinician wants to develop a treatment or an assessment protocol, a ready and often willing pool of subjects is available within an existing group program. When the clinician obtains a new assessment tool and needs some practice in administration of the instrument before giving the test in a standardized fashion, group members may provide the prerequisite practice experiences.

REFERENCES

1. Eisenson J. Adult Aphasia (2nd ed). Englewood Cliffs, NJ: Prentice Hall, 1983;1.
2. Avent J. Manual of Cooperative Group Treatment for Aphasia. Boston: Butterworth–Heinemann, 1997;1.
3. Batavia AL, DeJong G. Prospective payment for medical rehabilitation. The DHHS report to Congress. Arch Phys Med Rehabil 1988;69:377.
4. Beeson P, Holland AL. Aphasia Groups: An Approach to Long-term Rehabilitation. Telerounds #19. Tucson, AZ: National Center for Neurogenic Communication Disorders, 1994.
5. Elman R. Group Treatment of Neurogenic Communication Disorders: The Expert Clinician's View. Boston: Butterworth–Heinemann, 1999.
6. Brindley P, Copeland M, Demain C, Martyn P. A comparison of ten chronic Broca's aphasics following intensive and nonintensive periods of therapy. Aphasiology 1989;8:695.
7. Elman R, Bernstein-Ellis E, Beeson P, et al. Aphasia Groups: Who, What, When, Why. Paper presented at the American Speech-Language-Hearing Association Convention, Orlando, FL, December 1995.
8. Kearns K. Group Therapy for Aphasia: Theoretical and Practical Considerations. In R Chapey (ed), Language Intervention Strategies in Adult Aphasia (3rd ed). Baltimore: Williams & Wilkins, 1994;304.
9. Luterman DM. Counseling Persons with Communicative Disorders and Their Families (3rd ed). Austin, TX: Pro-Ed, 1996;111

10. Seligman M. Group Psychotherapy and Counseling with Special Populations. Baltimore: University Park, 1977;1.
11. Yalom ID. Theory and Practice of Group Psychotherapy (3rd ed). New York: HarperCollins, 1985;3.
12. Simmons-Mackie N, Damico J. Reformulating the definition of compensatory strategies in aphasia. Aphasiology 1997;11:761.
13. Brookshire R. An Introduction to Neurogenic Communication Disorders (3rd ed). Minneapolis: BRK, 1986;174.
14. Darley FL. Aphasia. Philadelphia: Saunders, 1982;264.
15. Davis GA. A Survey of Adult Aphasia and Related Language Disorders (2nd ed). Englewood Cliffs, NJ: Prentice Hall, 1993;287.
16. Schuell H, Jenkins JJ, Jiminez-Pabon J. Aphasia in Adults. New York: Harper & Row, 1964;343.
17. Aten J. Group therapy for aphasic patients: let's show it works. Aphasiology 1991;5:559.
18. Loverso F. Aphasia group therapy: a commentary. Aphasiology 1991;5:567.
19. Fawcus M. Group Therapy: A Learning Situation. In C Code, D Muller (eds), Aphasia Therapy. London: Edward Arnold, 1983;113.
20. Wertz RT, Collins MH, Weiss D, et al. Veterans Administration cooperative study on aphasia. A comparison of individual and group treatment. J Speech Hear Res 1981;24:580.
21. Elman RJ, Burnstein-Ellis E. Effectiveness of Group Communication Treatment for Individuals with Chronic Aphasia: Results on Communicative and Linguistic Measures. Paper presented at the Clinical Aphasiology Conference, Newport, RI, June 1996.
22. Avent J. Group treatment in aphasia using the cooperative learning method. J Med Speech-Lang Pathol 1997;5:9.
23. Marshall RC. Problem-focused group therapy for mildly aphasic clients. Am J Speech-Lang Pathol 1993;2:31.
24. Makenzie C. Four weeks of intensive therapy followed by four weeks of no treatment. Aphasiology 1991;5:435.
25. Aten J, Caliguri M, Holland A. The efficacy of functional communication therapy for chronic aphasic patients. J Speech Hear Disord 1972;47:93.
26. Bollinger R, Musson N, Holland A. A study of group communication intervention with chronically aphasic persons. Aphasiology 1993;7:301.
27. Shelton CF, Bakker K. Perceived Effectiveness of Group Treatment for Aphasia. Paper presented at the American Speech-Language-Hearing Association Convention, Boston, November 1997.
28. Bernstein J. A supportive group for spouses of stroke patients. Aphasia Apraxia Agnosia 1979;1:30.
29. Friedland J, McColl M. Social support for stroke survivors: development and evaluation of an intervention program. Phys Occup Ther Geriat 1989;7:55.
30. Kinsella G, Duffy FD. Psychosocial re-adjustments in the spouses of aphasic patients. Scand J Rehabil Med 1978;11:129.
31. Fratalli C. Quality Improvement. In R Lubinski, C Fratalli (eds), Professional Issues in Speech-Language Pathology and Audiology. San Diego: Singular, 1994;246.
32. Lubinski R. A Model for Intervention: Communication Skills, Effectiveness, and Opportunity. In B Shadden (ed), Communication Behavior and Aging. Baltimore: Williams & Wilkins, 1988;294.

33. Simmons-Mackie N. A solution to the discharge dilemma in aphasia: social approaches to aphasia management. Aphasiology 1998;12:231.

34. Kagan A, Gailey GF. Functional Is Not Enough: Training Conversation Partners for Aphasia Adults. In AL Holland, ML Forbes (eds), Aphasia Treatment: World Perspectives. London: Chapman & Hall, 1993;199.

35. Kagan A. Supported conversation for adults with aphasia. Aphasiology 1998; 12:816.

36. Kagan A. Revealing the competence of aphasic adults through conversation: a challenge to health professions. Top Stroke Rehabil 1995;2:15.

37. Lyon J. Communication use and participation in life for adults with aphasia in natural settings: the scope of the problem. Am J Speech-Lang Pathol 1992;1:7.

38. Pachalska M. Group therapy for aphasia patients. Aphasiology 1991;5:541.

39. Marshall RC. Problem-Solving Support Groups for Long-Term Brain I(in press).

40. Pachalska MK. Prevention of the state of social dependence of patients afflicted with aphasia. Am J Soc Psychiatry 1982;2:51.

41. Singler JK. The Stroke Group. In M Seligman (ed), Group Psychotherapy and Counseling with Special Populations. Baltimore: University Park, 1977;43.

42. Tonkovich J, Burke J. Managed Care's Impact on Services for Adult Neurogenic Communication Disorders. Paper presented at the American Speech-Language-Hearing Association Convention, New Orleans, November 1994.

43. Boysen AE, Wertz RT. Clinician costs in aphasia treatment: how much is a word worth? In M Lemme (ed), Clinical Aphasiology, 1996;24:207.

44. Warren RL, Gabriel C, Johnson A, Gaddie A. Efficacy During Acute Rehabilitation. In R Brookshire (ed), Clinical Aphasiology Conference Proceedings. Minneapolis: BRK, 1987;1.

45. Busch C. Functional outcome: reimbursement issues. In M Lemme (ed), Clinical Aphasiology. Austin, TX: Pro-Ed, 1993;21:73.

46. Elman RJ. Aphasia Treatment Planning in an Outpatient Medical Rehabilitation Center: Where Do We Go from Here? Division 2 Newsletter. American Speech-Language-Hearing Association 1994;4:9.

47. Marshall RC. Aphasia treatment in the early postonset period: managing our resources effectively. Am J Speech-Lang Pathol 1997;6:5.

48. Logemann JA. Creativity Plus Activism Equals a Formula for Managing Change. Presidential address presented at American Speech-Language-Hearing Association Convention, New Orleans, November 1994;27.

49. Fawcus M. Managing group therapy: further considerations. Aphasiology 1991;5:555.

50. Nash LN, Lubinski R. Effective In-Service Training for Staff Working with Communication-Impaired Patients. In R Lubinski (ed), Dementia and Communication. San Diego: Singular, 1995;279.

51. Ricco-Schwartz S. Fostering an empathic approach: an in-service curriculum for nonmedical professionals, paraprofessionals, and families of aphasic patients. Gerontol Geriatr Educ 1992;2:58.

52. Hunt MI. A Social Language Group for Aphasics. In R Brookshire (ed), Clinical Aphasiology Conference Proceedings. Minneapolis: BRK, 1974;138.

53. Mogil S, Bloom D, Gray L, Lefkowitz N. A Unique Method for the Follow-Up of Aphasic Patients. In R Brookshire (ed), Clinical Aphasiology Conference Proceedings. Minneapolis: BRK, 1978;314.

3

Logistics

A song about little things meaning a lot was popular several years ago. If you are starting a group, this tune is a good one to hum. The success or the failure of a program may depend on logistics, which really constitutes many little things. For example, the clinician-manager who must continually spend his or her time resolving transportation issues for group patients will soon lose enthusiasm for the group work. The emphasis of this chapter is on attending to the details, large and small, that promote running successful group therapy programs.

RECRUITMENT

You need to know whether the health care organization, clinic, your community speech center, or private practice can attract enough patients to support and sustain a group. Different recruiting tactics are necessary for groups sponsored by larger (e.g., hospitals), smaller (e.g., community centers), and long-term care facilities (e.g., nursing homes).

Large Organizations

Larger organizations (e.g., hospitals) have many clinics, programs, and services that are potential recruitment sources for group treatment participants. Primary care and specialty (e.g., stroke, neurology, dementia, and movement disorders) clinics are one source of capturing patients. The speech-language pathologist might be monitoring the communication status of patients in these clinics to document changes in communicative status or to assist in the diagnoses of communication disorders.

Make sure to establish, develop, and nurture working relationships with physicians and nurses who staff these clinics. Keep them informed about changes in patients' communicative status that suggest group treatment may be viable. Be sure that these referral sources understand that patients with aphasia and related disorders can make progress even when their deficits are chronic.[1–3] Physicians and nurses can be alerted to a patient's "potential" to benefit from group work by a chart note that tells (1) what the patient is doing that makes him or her a group candidate, (2) how group treatment will benefit the patient, and (3) the cost and duration of group treatment. An example chart note is provided in Figure 3.1.

The rehabilitation team plays a vital role in the group referral process. Concurrence, cooperation, and coordination are the operative words for successful teams.[4] The team decides when treatment should begin, what kind of treatment is needed, how much treatment the patient will receive, where treatment will take place, and how long it will last. Team members (i.e., physician, social worker, occupational therapist, physical therapist, recreational therapist, neuropsychologist, and speech-language pathologist) can do much to promote the use of group treatment. No longer do rehabilitation teams adhere to tradition. Capitation models of payment in which a fixed amount of money is given on a per-person basis regardless of the number of services rendered requires the team to focus not only on what is best for the patient, but what is least costly to the system. When resources are limited, excessive or unnecessary services provided to one patient may deny another basic care.[5] One of the more important team functions may be deciding when group treatment is an equally valuable, but less costly alternative to individual treatment.

Counseling and patient education are required by the Joint Commission of Accreditation of Healthcare Organizations.[6] These programs, also mentioned in the preceding chapter, involve patient education activities of physicians, nurses, dietitians, and other providers. Health care organizations also have more generic and general education offerings. Examples include wellness and fitness programs to teach about exercise, stress, diet, and other health-enhancing regimes. Cardiac rehabilitation and smoking cessation programs are commonplace and also included in most health care packages. Some organizations sponsor chapters of Alcoholics Anonymous. All educational programs are fertile recruiting ground. The clinician-manager should apprise the individuals responsible for these programs of group treatment opportunities.

Community-based educational seminars are sometimes offered by larger health care organizations. Selected seminars might provide information about stroke, diabetes, cancer, and Alzheimer's disease. Some health care organizations coordinate these public information efforts with nonprofit agencies (e.g., American Heart Association) and use the program as a marketing tool to attract customers. Clinician-managers

Background information: Mr. E., a 57-year-old, right-handed, married contractor, had a left-hemisphere stroke with resulting Broca's aphasia and right-sided weakness 9 months ago. Speech-language pathology has been following Mr. E. since his dismissal from individual treatment at 3 months postonset.

Subjective: The patient and his wife have a large circle of friends. Mr. E. has been reluctant to reinvolve himself in former social activities that he and his wife enjoyed before the stroke. This has frustrated Mrs. E., who reports that she will look into alternative living arrangements for her husband unless things can be improved. There appear to be no physical or cognitive reasons why Mr. E. cannot resume activities, such as playing poker, going to the casino, attending weekly potlucks, and going to church, other than that he is embarrassed about his slow, laborious speech and word-finding difficulties.

Objective: Today's follow-up visit shows that Mr. E. has significantly improved his ability to "get his ideas across" since stopping individual treatment. He does this by supplementing meager verbalizations with gestures, writing, and drawing. Knowledgeable partners, specifically his wife and the therapist, readily understand his communications. For example, he communicated that his 26-year-old son had moved to Atlanta, Georgia, to take a job with Delta Airlines.

Assessment: Mr. E should expand his repertoire of conversational partners and develop confidence in his now emerging ability to communicate his thoughts. Mrs. E. is sufficiently concerned about a nonexistent social life that she may divorce her husband and/or place him in less independent living situation. Group treatment will help Mr. E. in this regard and permit him to further develop use of his compensatory communication skills socially.

Plan: (1) Enroll Mr. E. in weekly group treatment in 2 weeks' time. (2) Over the 2-week waiting period, have wife keep a log of all social activities engaged in to provide a pretreatment baseline measure. (3) Monitor social activity over a 6-month period of weekly group treatment. (4) Have wife complete ASHA-FACS at the beginning of the group treatment period and at 2-month intervals.

Figure 3.1 Example of a chart note that alerts the physician to the need for group treatment for a patient with Broca's aphasia. (ASHA-FACS = American Speech-Language-Hearing Association Functional Assessment of Communication Skills.)

recruiting patients for group treatment should consider becoming a part of the seminar program. If presenting seminars is not possible, a brief announcement about the availability of group therapy in the material handed out at a seminar may be helpful.

Regular family support groups are sponsored by health care organization and nonprofit agencies (e.g., Alzheimer's Association). Stroke clubs, often under the auspices of the American Heart Association, are found in many communities.[7] Community support groups assist families in coping with the long-term residuals of disabilities secondary to stroke, brain trauma, and progressive diseases. They provide stroke and traumatic brain injury survivors with opportunities for socialization, as well as exchanging information among persons in similar circumstances. Because these groups have open public meetings, the clinician-manager or a member of the rehabilitation staff may want to attend a meeting or two to market group treatment availability. In addition, the clinician-manager who wants to start a group program should make this fact known to the National Aphasia Association (NAA; P.O. Box 1887, Murray Hill Station, New York, NY 10156-0611), a clearinghouse for information on aphasia and related disorders. He or she should ensure that the NAA has appropriate identifying information to give to persons who are new to the area or who may be seeking therapeutic assistance.

Small Programs

Recruiting group therapy patients for smaller programs (e.g., community centers, university clinics, and speech and hearing centers) requires different strategies. Although the clinician-manager working in a larger medical center has many in-house sites from which to recruit group patients, those who wish to start a group treatment program in a community-based clinic do not. Clinicians who desire to start a group treatment in a small community center or clinic need different recruitment strategies. Visiting ongoing support groups and making a pitch for group treatment is an effective strategy. The NAA is also a referral source.

The major source for recruitment of group patients for community clinics, however, is speech-language pathologists in private practice or those who work in settings where group therapy is not available. How to make these interpersonal contacts will depend on individual circumstances. Potential ways of marketing a group treatment program include making telephone calls, attending state meetings, hosting and attending professional education programs, and mailing periodic announcements. Informative speeches to service clubs on stroke and stroke rehabilitation may also facilitate recruitment. Finally, direct advertising in local newspapers or writing a brief article on aphasia for local publication should not be ruled out.

Long-Term Care Programs

If you work in a long-term care facility, recruitment is not a major issue. Nursing homes, retirement centers, adult day care centers, and residential programs have all the patients they need to create groups.[8] Of course, many logistic and other issues must be dealt with in starting groups in long-term care facilities, but recruitment is not one of them.

For the clinician-manager thinking about starting a group in a long-term care setting, the biggest obstacle to recruitment is making the effort. The second might be what to do once this effort is made. The clinician-manager may find, as Forrest Gump said, "Life is like a box of chocolates. You never know what you're going to get." Approximately one million persons are living with the residual effects of a stroke at any given time, and approximately 400,000 head injuries occur each year.[9, 10] The clinician-manager who begins to recruit patients for a group may discover that he or she has uncovered the tip of an iceberg and that a shortage of clients to participate in group treatment programs does not exist.

TRANSPORTATION ISSUES

Many brain-injured patients do not drive. Others may drive but consciously restrict where and when they drive. Some nondrivers have private transportation, usually provided by an SO; some do not. Often a patient believes that he or she has an available source of transportation, but this source is not reliable. Transportation can be a logistic nightmare for the clinician and patient alike on days that groups meet. A successful group treatment program requires clinician-managers who are creative and decisive in solving transportation problems.

Nondrivers

The nondriver without an SO to bring him or her to and from group therapy probably relies on public transportation. If the patient cannot ride the city bus unassisted, he or she can use handicapped transportation services (e.g., lifts or wheelchair vans). For these patients, reliable transportation is paramount. These individuals may seldom leave home. The weekly group session may be the highlight of their week.[11, 12] If not picked up or picked up late, patients are unable to attend or arrive late for group, causing them to become frustrated and discouraged.

Nondriving patients must sometimes wait to be picked up or returned home. Handicapped ride services are often over-scheduled; their timeliness is affected by weather and other uncontrollable factors (e.g., heavy traffic). The clinician should forewarn patients of the possibilities. Showing some appreciation and goodwill may facilitate cooperation of handicapped transportation services. Establish a personal contact with a responsible individual, preferably the dispatcher and schedule persons. Let them know how much you appreciate their efforts on the part of the patient and how important group therapy is to the patient.

Some nondriving brain-injured patients and patients with minimal physical disabilities can learn to ride the bus.[13] In this case, the clinician-manager should be sure that the patient is able to travel from the bus stop to the group treatment area safely. If the location of the bus stop requires crossing a busy street, negotiating several steps, or walking through an unsafe area, riding the bus may be a problem. Look into these issues.

A patient with slow reaction times, poor judgment, or attentional difficulties may assert that he or she can ride the bus. Make sure the patient has the ability to ride the bus before advising use of public transportation. When ability is suspect, consider recruiting an escort for the patient from volunteer services or having a fellow group member accompany the patient from the bus stop to the treatment area rather than abandoning outright the possibility of using the bus.

When the group member is a nondriver and another person provides the transportation, the major logistic problem is parking. If the person being transported has physical limitations, parking should be available relatively close to the treatment area. Often, the patient (i.e., person being transported) is dropped at the door of the facility, and the driver parks the car. In some cases, the patient may need some assistance until the driver has parked the vehicle and can escort the patient to the group meeting area. If the patient arrives by taxi, similar circumstances occur. One way to solve this problem is to enlist the aid of a hospital volunteer to escort taxi-driven patients to the treatment area or monitor the patient until the driver parks the vehicle.

Drivers

Group patients who drive themselves to treatment must also deal with logistic issues, specifically parking, scheduling, and planning of their driving route to be on time for group meetings. When appropriate, handicapped parking permits should be issued. If a patient is not eligible for a permanent handicapped license plate, the institution can issue a temporary handicapped parking permit for the group treatment session. Some brain-injured persons restrict their driving to nonpeak hours, and this should be considered when scheduling group sessions. Patients who drive to group meetings should be cautioned to leave early when delays due to weather, construction, and special event traffic are anticipated. Those attending group for the first time need a good map to guide them to and from the treatment site. When possible, advise the a new member to make a practice run before the first group meeting. Teach group patients who drive to therapy about riding the bus. The bus gives them a backup system if, for some reason, they are unable to drive themselves.

Transportation Costs

Many stroke survivors are on fixed incomes. The cost of transportation to group treatment is not a part of their budget, especially when the individual lives some distance from the program. Know the eligibility and other requirements governing free or discounted handicapped transportation: senior citizen discounts, handicapped passes, monthly passes, or discounts for riding the bus during non–prime-time hours. Become familiar with the available options for public and private transportation in the area. This information can be summarized in a handout to be given to prospective group patients. In some instances, the clinician-manager may want to write a letter verifying the necessity and importance of transportation assistance in bringing the patient to treatment.

The use of a volunteer driver for group patients should also be considered. If family members are unavailable, senior citizens, members of service organizations, and others may provide patient transportation for a small fee. Group members living near each other may benefit by forming a carpool. If only one group member is capable of driving, passengers (i.e., the other group members) can reimburse the driver for gas money. A benefit of collaborative transportation ventures is that they afford group members added opportunities for socialization and communicative interaction, such as having coffee before the meeting or going to lunch after.

Independence Issues

Some therapeutic benefits are derived when a group member can travel to and from the group session without any assistance from the

SO. It is a step toward independence for the patient. For some, the trip to and from the clinic is an adventure. They meet people. They are forced to do some communicating. It gives them something to talk about. Moreover, riding the bus or taking the handicapped lift takes time. The patient's primary caregiver will have a few hours of welcome respite to focus on other tasks, to rest, and to revitalize him- or herself.

SPACE

Long ago, the space and planning criteria for speech and audiology clinics in Veterans Administration hospitals made provisions for group treatment space. One room was assigned to speech pathology for aphasia therapy; a second was assigned to audiology for the purposes of aural rehabilitation. Although having assigned space underscored the role of group treatment in the 1945 postwar era, assigned space for group treatment is an unheard-of luxury today. To find space for your group, you may need to do some looking around. Begin with a walking tour of your facility. Find out if a conference, activity, multipurpose, or other room that will be a suitable space for group treatment is available. Identify the individual responsible for scheduling events in that room and "suck up" to him or her. Negotiate the use of this space with the understanding that it will not be your space but that it will be shared by many programs and components of the organization. Make sure any commitments for use of space at certain times are put in writing.

Group Room Features

The group room must be handicapped-accessible, quiet, well ventilated, and properly lit. If possible, the room should be near handicapped-accessible bathrooms and a waiting area for family members. Room size is a consideration. If your only option is a room that limits growth, plan to develop additional groups. Some general-purpose rooms could actually be too large. If a room is too large, consider asking management to install a retractable room divider or use movable partitions to make the space more intimate and conducive to therapy activities. If that is not possible, make do. Larger is better than too small or no room at all.

Furnishings and Equipment

The furnishings and equipment needed in the group treatment room depend on the composition of the group. Patients with severe communicative deficits need to sit at a table so they can use drawing and writing to supplement limited verbal skills. The table supports the use of augmentative communication aids used by many of these patients in therapy. If a table is used, it should be of sufficient height to accommodate wheelchairs. Round tables are preferred because they facilitate eye contact and interaction among group members, and they are less formal than rectangular arrangements. If a round table is not available, move three rectangular tables into a U-shaped arrangement. Chairs should be sturdy, shallow-backed, and of adequate height to allow the patient to sit comfortably and stand up easily. Casters on the chairs are not recommended because of the possibility of a patient falling when trying to sit in a chair that rolls away. A table is not necessary when group members use verbal communication as their only means of interacting. Additionally, little writing and no use of augmentative systems are needed during the session. In this case, a circular seating arrangement works best. Chairs should be comfortable but not too deep, because some patients may have difficulty getting in and out of them. All chairs should be identical so that no conflict occurs as to who sits where.

Certain props are useful in conducting a group session. Each room should have a wall-mounted erasable board so that patients can use writing and drawing options or the group leader can highlight certain points for the group's consideration. Additional props that might be useful include books, stimulus pictures (e.g., old movie stars), paper, pencils, crayons, clipboards, flip charts, a road atlas, maps, and name tags for group members. This list should not be considered exclusive.

More sophisticated equipment (e.g., computers, art supplies, and construction materials) and materials needed in the group area will largely depend on the composition and activities of the group. The clinician may want to use a videocassette recorder to record the meetings to present information to the group. Slide and overhead projectors may be used for some groups. Usually, the clinician will be allowed to leave these materials in the group room. Transporting materials and equipment to and from the group room for each meeting is time-consuming. Time is also wasted when the clinician leaves something critical to the group session back at the office. This problem can be solved by having a locked storage cabinet in the room for storage of necessary materials and equipment. Again, storage space should be negotiated with other users of the space.

Scheduling and Maintaining Space

Some group members become embarrassed when they arrive to find another meeting in progress in "their" group room. Get to know the person responsible for scheduling meeting rooms. Secure advance written confirmation of your group meeting at a specific time each week. Post the schedule of group meetings on the door outside the room. Put a sign that reads "Therapy in session" or "In use" on the door during the group meeting.

After the meeting, put the room back in order. Make sure that group members pick up after themselves. Erase the board. Return equipment to its proper location. If chairs and tables have been moved, return them to their designated locations. If other meetings precede your scheduled group session, inform group members that this space is shared and warn them not to "stick their heads in the door early" and disturb users of the "shared space." Exit the room promptly at the end of the meeting, particularly when another group meeting is scheduled after yours. If a situation arises when your group is displaced or moved because of an "emergency," be cooperative and congenial. Move your group to another space with a smile. A little courtesy will go far in ensuring that the group has a place to meet every week.

Meeting Times and Cancellations

Meeting with your group at an optimum time is not always feasible. Optimum times are 10:00 or 11:00 AM for older patients who prefer to travel to treatment at nonpeak traffic hours. For younger patients who might be working, 5:00 or 6:00 PM may work best. This schedule allows the patient time to get to the group after work and still get home for dinner. Often, patients attending group after work need a snack. One important factor in scheduling a group meeting is not making any changes (i.e., keep the time consistent).

Establish a policy for canceling group sessions. Bad weather is the most common reason for cancellation. Decide which conditions of inclement weather will cause the group session to be canceled automatically. One rule of thumb might be that when the public schools are closed because of bad weather, the group will not meet. Make sure group members and their families understand the policy.

If the meeting must be canceled because the clinician will be absent, let the group know this well in advance. Give the group a written reminder to avoid having patients show up for group sessions when you are not there. If the clinician will be absent on short notice, use a telephone tree. Member A calls member B; member B then calls member C; and so forth. This method avoids having a clinician, secretary, or colleague call each group member, and it promotes communication among group members.

SOME FINAL THOUGHTS

Clinicians and clinician-managers may need to spend a substantial amount of time on logistic operations: recruitment, solving transportation problems, obtaining space and equipment, scheduling, and establishing policies. Be flexible when first starting a group until all bugs are worked out. When you believe that things are working well, *do not make any changes*, unless absolutely necessary. Maintaining the same routine is important for two reasons: (1) Changes require development of a new logistic plan, and (2) brain-injured persons appreciate the routine of a schedule.

REFERENCES

1. Bollinger R, Musson N, Holland A. A study of group communication intervention with chronically aphasic persons. Aphasiology 1993;7:301.
2. Aten J, Caliguri M, Holland A. The efficacy of functional communication therapy for chronic aphasic patients. J Speech Hear Disord 1982;47:93.
3. Marshall RC. Problem-Solving Support Groups for Long-Term Brain Injured Adults. Paper presented at the American Speech-Language-Hearing Association Convention, Boston, November 1997.
4. Golper LA. Sourcebook for Medical Speech Pathology. San Diego: Singular, 1993;4.
5. Frattali CM. Clinical Care in a Changing Health Care System. In N Helm-Estabrooks, A Holland (eds), Approaches to Treatment of Aphasia. San Diego: Singular, 1997;241.
6. Joint Commission on Accreditation of Healthcare Organizations. Agenda for Change. Oakbrook Terrace, IL: Joint Commission on Accreditation of Healthcare Organizations, 1987;1.
7. Sanders S, Hamby EI, Nelson M. You Are Not Alone. Nashville: American Heart Association, 1984;6.
8. Singler JK. The Stroke Group. In M Seligman (ed), Group Psychotherapy and Counseling with Special Populations. Baltimore: University Park Press, 1982;43.
9. Kurtzke J. Epidemiology of Cerebrovascular Disease. In Cerebrovascular Survey Report for Joint Council Subcommittee on Cerebrovascular Disease. Washington, DC: National Institute of Neurological and Communication Disorders and Stroke, and National Heart and Lung Institute, 1980;23.
10. Grossman RG, Gildenberg PI. Head Injury: Basic and Clinical Concepts. New York: Raven Press, 1982;33.
11. Beeson P, Holland A. Aphasia Groups: An Approach to Long-Term Rehabilitation. Telerounds #19. Tucson, AZ: National Center for Neurogenic Communication Disorders, 1994.
12. Springer O. Facilitating group rehabilitation. Aphasiology 1991;5:563.
13. Marshall RC. Documentation Strategies in Medical Speech Pathology: Seizing the Moment. Short Course. Seattle: American Speech-Language-Hearing Association, 1996.

4

Funding

This chapter (1) presents cost estimates for group therapy, (2) discusses the value of group therapy for aphasia in relation to individual therapy, and (3) offers suggestions for obtaining funds to provide group therapy for patients with aphasia who are not covered for this service by a health care plan. Until recently, clinicians have been relatively unconcerned about costs of their services. The restructuring of the health care system may bring about staff reductions, limits in the amount of treatment patients with aphasia can receive, and less costly treatment paradigms.[1, 2] Restructuring may be a "boon" to group therapy if this method can be shown to have value to the health care system. Value is defined as the relationship between the result of the care and its cost.[2] Value is discussed in more detail later.

COST OF GROUP TREATMENT

Return to the scenario depicted for the Paul Broca Medical Center (PBMC) in Chapter 3. Imagine that the PBMC has now seen the error of its ways. Its chief executive officer, DeRenzi Lotharo, is unhappy about the number of stroke patients who have opted to obtain their medical care at the Carl Wernicke Medical Center because it has a group treatment program for aphasia. He wants some "bottom line" figures for starting a group program at PBMC.

Speech Pathology Unit Costs

PBMC has four speech-language pathologists (SLPs) on its staff. The names, amount of experience, and yearly salaries of these clinicians are provided in Table 4.1. These salaries are based on estimates approximating what SLPs are paid at the GS-13, GS-12, GS-11, and GS-9 levels in Veterans Administration (VA) medical centers. Total salary dollars

Table 4.1
Speech-language pathology unit costs to the Paul Broca Medical Center.

Staff Member	Experience	Level	Yearly Salary ($)
Sally Schuell, Mgr.	10 years	GS-13	60,000
Edgar Eisenson	5 years	GS-12	50,000
Hillary Holland	2 years	GS-11	43,000
Mack Simmons	CFY	GS-9	37,000
Line 1 (total salary)			$190,000
Line 2 (fringe benefits: line 1 × .27)			$51,300
Line 3 (overhead costs: line 1 × .20)			$38,000
Line 4 (total budget: line 1 + 2 + 3)			$279,300
Line 5 (average cost per SLP: line 4/4)			$69,825
Line 6 (costs per hour of service: line 5/2,080)			$33.56

CFY = clinical fellowship year; SLP = speech-language pathologist.

for the PBMC speech pathology unit are shown in line 1 of Table 4.1. PBMC has a good benefits package. This includes health care, a 401K plan, and stock options in the parent company, Horatio Alger Health Enterprises. Benefits are calculated at 27% of the employee's salary. This information is given on line 2 of the table. Overhead costs associated with the operation of the speech-language pathology unit include utilities, equipment, supplies, building maintenance, computer services, staff education, and clerical support. These costs have been calculated as 20% of the employee's salary and are shown in line 3 of Table 4.1. The total budget for the speech pathology unit is shown in line 4.

The next step is to determine the average yearly cost of each SLP to PBMC by dividing the total budget by the number of employees—four. This figure is given on line 5 of Table 4.1. The last step is to determine an hourly cost of a SLP to PBMC. A work year contains 2,080 hours (52 weeks × 40 hours). The hourly figure is derived by dividing the average salary by 2,080 or $33.56, as shown on line 6 of Table 4.1.

Estimating Group Treatment Charges

Now that we have an approximate estimate of what PBMC spends for 1 hour of an SLP's time, we can move on to determining a cost for 1 hour of group treatment. Here I will explore fee-for-service and managed care scenarios. Let us assume that PBMC charges $165 per hour

Table 4.2
Profits and losses for the Paul Broca Medical Center resulting from 1 hour of
group treatment under fee-for-service and managed care scenarios.

	Number	Cost per Patient ($)	Profit/Loss
Fee for service ($165)			
Full	4	165	+660 (597)
50%	4	83	+332 (269)
25%	4	41	+165 (102)
10%	4	17	+68 (5)
Capitation ($100)			
Full	4	100	+400 (337)
50%	4	50	+200 (137)
25%	4	25	+100 (37)
10%	4	10	+40 (–23)
Salary equivalency ($50)			
Full	4	50	+200 (137)
50%	4	25	+100 (37)
25%	4	13	+52 (–10)
10%	4	5	+20 (–43)

Note: Figures are based on a group of four patients. Dollar amounts in parentheses
represent the subtraction of 2 hours of a speech-language pathologist's time
($63.22). All figures rounded to nearest dollar.

for speech and language therapy. Although treatment charges vary
widely across the United States, $165 is the amount that PVAMC paid
per hour of treatment delivered to patients not seen at the hospital.
The number sticks with me because I, and the rest of the staff, were
responsible for monitoring the expenditure of these funds. Therefore,
fairly or unfairly, I used this figure for the calculations in Table 4.2.
Although the cost of the SLP's time remains the same regardless of the
charges billed, I took the liberty of doubling this cost for an hour of
group treatment to include time spent in planning and documentation.
Planning and documentation time has been figured into all group treatment calculations in Table 4.2. All calculations are based on groups of
four persons.

Table 4.2 shows that for 1 hour of speech and language therapy at
the $165 rate, PBMC makes $131.44 ($165 – $33.56)—a little more
than 300%. This amount is not bad, but perhaps it is a little high. Also,
this amount is an individual treatment charge, and this book is about
group treatment. Clinicians and clinician-managers who want to start

a group should think about what the appropriate charge is for this service *before* approaching their administrations with a plan. This charge should allow the organization, in this case PBMC, to make a profit, but reflect a cost savings to the payer. The upper third of Table 4.2 gives approximate group treatment revenues for PBMC using a fee-for-service model. Here we see that if charges for group treatment are billed at the same rate as those for individual treatment, PBMC will earn a good profit. If group treatment is billed at 50%, 25%, and 10% of individual treatment charges, PBMC will still make money, but not as much.

Because all indications are that fee-for-service payment plans have seen better days, the middle third of Table 4.2 examines group treatment charges in a capitation model.[1–4] Assume that PBMC can only charge $100 per hour for speech and language therapy—or even worse, only $50, $25, or $10. Table 4.2 shows that in three of four of these scenarios, PBMC will still make a profit on group treatment.

The lower third of Table 4.2 also estimates group treatment charges using a salary equivalency model. The $50 charge approximates what Medicare will pay for aphasia treatment under this model. Under this system of salary equivalency, group treatment will be profitable to PBMC at the $50 rate and even at a rate of $25. Only if group treatment charges were less than $13 would PBMC lose money.

Of course, no health care organization should have to suffer a loss. So how might PBMC keep the cost of group treatment relatively low but still make a profit? One strategy would be to have five, six, or more patients in the group—not an uncommon practice for groups for mildly aphasic clients.[5] Another would be to have some of the preparation, data keeping, and record keeping done by a student trainee, a volunteer supervised by an SLP, or a speech-language pathology assistant. The point is that deciding how a group treatment program can be profitable can be flexible. Perhaps the most important responsibility of the clinician-manager is to create a win-win situation. This outlook involves determining what is fair and equitable for payer, patient, and provider.

Determining Value

As stated earlier, value reflects a relationship between the result of the care and its cost.[2] One way to show the value of group treatment is to conduct a study that shows aphasic patients improve as much with group as individual treatment, but that group treatment costs less. The value of group treatment is clearly illustrated by the results of the 1981 VA Cooperative Study on Aphasia.[6] In this multicenter study, patients with aphasia meeting strict selection criteria were randomly assigned to group A, individual treatment, or to group B, group treatment. All patients received 8 hours of treatment per week during the time they were enrolled in the study. Group A patients received 4 hours of individual stimulus-response treatment in all communicative modalities (e.g., comprehension, speaking, reading, and writing tasks scored correct or incorrect) supplemented by 4 hours of machine-assisted treatment (e.g., speech and language drills) per week. Group B patients received 4 hours of group treatment (three to seven members per group) designed to enhance the use of language in a social setting (e.g., group discussion of current events and topics) supplemented by 4 hours of recreational activities (e.g., field trips to a museum) per week.

All patients were evaluated with a battery of speech, language, and neurologic tests at intake (4 weeks) and every 11 weeks thereafter, up to 48 weeks postonset. Results showed that both groups improved significantly over the course of the study. However, differences between the groups were few and those that did occur were confined to performance on the Porch Index of Communicative Ability (PICA),[7] particularly the writing subtests. Only patients receiving individual treatment worked on writing in therapy.

Two critical factors in the VA study set it apart from other investigations of group treatment. The first is that patients entered the study at 4 weeks postonset. The second is that no patient had received prior speech and language treatment. These factors are important in thinking about "value," because most group studies have been carried out with chronic aphasic patients who had prior individual treatment or were receiving individual treatment concurrently with group treatment.[5, 8-10] The VA study thus provides a model for analyzing group treatment results in relation to the aforementioned definition of "value."

The calculations derived in Table 4.3 are based on data from the VA cooperative study. These show the mean overall PICA percentiles for 24 patients in group A (i.e., individual treatment) and 25 patients in group B (i.e., group treatment) at the 26-week evaluation. At 4 weeks postonset, the mean overall PICA percentile for group A patients was 46.04; the mean for group B patients was 46.32. After 22 weeks of treatment, the mean overall PICA percentile for group A patients was 69.96 and 62.96 for group B.

Table 4.3 shows the approximate cost of providing group and individual treatment to patients in the VA Cooperative Study using current cost figures. Each patient was treated for 8 hours per week for 22 weeks. Therefore, each patient received 176 hours of treatment (8×22). The cost of this treatment is obtained by multiplying 176 by the average per hour salary for a SLP ($\$33.56 \times 176 = \$5,906.56$). The cost of treating four individual patients over the same time period ($\$33.56 \times 176 \times 4 = \$23,626.24$) would be quadrupled. In a group of four patients, the amount of time and cost would be equivalent to that of a single individual. In this well-controlled study, group treatment was obviously less

Table 4.3
Estimated costs in 1998 dollars of group and individual treatment based on
information from the 1981 Veterans Administration cooperative study.

	Group A (Individual)	Group B (Group)
Mean PICA overall percentile		
intake	46.04	46.32
22 weeks	69.96	62.96
Hours in treatment per patient	176	176
Cost per hour ($)	33.56	33.56
Cost per patient ($)	5,906.56	1,476.64
Cost for four patients ($)	23,626.24	5,906.56

PICA = Porch Index of Communicative Ability.

costly, and it achieved equivalent results to individual treatment as measured by the PICA. In this scenario, group treatment may have had
more value because equivalent results were obtained at a lesser cost.

FUNDING SOURCES

Some patients with aphasia have no funds to cover group treatment.
When therapy is still warranted and funds to cover it are not available,
alternatives to dismissal are available if clinician-managers and clinicians are willing to seek them out.

Most medical institutions have tax-exempt foundations. Large
health care organizations have nonprofit foundations that receive mil-
lions of dollars to support research and other worthwhile programs.
Often, these moneys are gifts from grateful patients. Foundations host
fundraising events of all types. Consider approaching the foundation
associated with your organization about earmarking a sum of money
for group treatment for patients with aphasia who cannot afford it.
Similarly, if the health care system in which you work is a nonprofit
organization, it will assume the responsibilities of caring for the indi-
gent and absorb the losses. Ask your administration about funding
some scholarships for patients to receive group treatment.

The clinician-manager may want to consider asking a local service
club (e.g., Seratoma Foundation, Lions, Kiwanis, Rotary, Elks Clubs)
to sponsor a patient with aphasia for group treatment. These organizations like to help. If they do help, let the club membership know how

much their help means. A brief presentation at a meeting of a service club to share how their generosity betters the lives of individual patients may be all that is required by the clinician-manager to gain a sponsor for group treatment.

Another funding source is corporations and affluent individuals. Ask them about sponsoring a patient's group treatment. Do not rule out organizing your own fundraising events. Consider walk-a-thons, theater nights, and other events that provide scholarships for persons who cannot afford group treatment. These events also will raise public awareness of the long-term consequences of aphasia. Although the group treatment charge may be beyond the patient's budget, the clinician-manager could ask the patient to pay part of the cost as a copayment. It may also be possible to have a sliding scale for group payments based on the patient's income. Installment payment plans are another alternative.

Clinicians fully realize that the consequences of aphasia and related sequelae are long-term but that with continued effort, patients will improve. When the funds for rehabilitation are truly exhausted, consider giving some of your time. The concept of "service" suggests a willingness to give and to give freely to help someone else. Many people give of their time to the less fortunate within their churches, clubs, and communities. The willingness to extend one's self for the benefit of another, according to Peck,[11] epitomizes the nature of love. What does an hour or two of professional time from a SLP supported by his or her employing institution really cost?

REFERENCES

1. Frattali CM. Clinical Care in a Changing Health System. In N Helm-Estabrooks, A Holland (eds), Approaches to the Treatment of Aphasia. San Diego: Singular, 1997;241.
2. Warren RL. Outcome measurement: moving toward the patient. SID 2 Newsletter 1996;6:5.
3. Frattali CM. Measuring disability. SID 2 Newsletter 1996;6:7.
4. Hecht JS, Tonkovich JD. Rehabilitation Funding. In GL Wallace (ed), Adult Aphasia Rehabilitation. Boston: Butterworth–Heinemann, 1996;21.
5. Marshall RC. Problem-focused group treatment for clients with mild aphasia. Am J Speech-Lang Pathol 1993;2:31.
6. Porch BE. Porch Index of Communicative Ability. Palo Alto, CA: Consulting Psychologists, 1981.
7. Wertz RT, Collins MH, Weiss D, et al. Veterans Administration cooperative study on aphasia. A comparison of individual and group treatment. J Speech Hear Res 1981;24:580.
8. Elman RJ, Burnstein-Ellis E. Effectiveness of Group Communication Treatment for Individuals with Chronic Aphasia: Results on Communicative and Lin-

guistic Measures. Paper presented at the Clinical Aphasiology Conference, Newport, RI, June 1996.

9. Bollinger R, Musson N, Holland A. A study of group communication intervention with chronically aphasic persons. Aphasiology 1993;7:301.

10. Aten J, Caliguri M, Holland A. The efficacy of functional communication therapy for chronic aphasic patients. J Speech Hear Disord 1982;47:93.

11. Peck S. The Road Less Traveled. New York: Simon & Schuster, 1973;84.

5

Group Composition

SIZE

A formula for determining the optimum size of a group has not been developed. Groups of four or five patients have been suggested by some writers.[1] Others have suggested that groups can be larger, particularly when they are discussion groups rather than groups that work on specific speech-language activities.[2] Groups can number as few as two in cooperative group treatment to 10 or more in problem-focused groups.[3-4] A group should not be so large that all members do not have a chance to participate or so small that group cohesiveness suffers when members are absent.[5] Four- to six-member groups are probably the norm. Groups can become too large; one of my groups once swelled to 12 members. When the possibility of splitting the group into two separate groups was discussed, group members protested that they knew each other well and often did things together (e.g., had lunch). Their cohesiveness made splitting the group into two smaller units difficult. These incidents can be avoided by making an a priori determination on optimal group size and sticking to it. As a group nears its maximum allowable size, develop a waiting list as additional group candidates are referred. When recruitment is ongoing, a second group can soon be started and allowed to grow on its own.

GROUP HOMOGENEITY

In homogenous groups, members share common features and attributes. Homogenous groups tend to achieve cohesiveness sooner than heterogeneous groups do, because they enable members to provide more immediate support for one another.[5, 6] Homogenous groups may be easier to manage and require less planning time than do heterogeneous groups. Consequently, the clinician can use the allotted treatment time more productively. Remember, however, that homogenous group members are not "clones" and that a homogenous group is also heterogeneous and diverse in many ways.[5] Factors that clinician-managers should consider in attempting to create homogenous groups include etiology, symptomatology, severity, age, and gender.

Etiology

Including brain-injured patients with dissimilar etiologies in the same group can be difficult.[7, 8] For example, stroke patients frequently fear having a second stroke, whereas younger traumatic brain injury (TBI) patients have little concern for this problem. Patients with physical handicaps are more concerned with walking than talking. Most clinicians remember the problems that occurred when younger patients with cognitive-communicative deficits were placed in vocational rehabilitation programs intended to serve the needs of mentally challenged individuals. These types of vocational rehabilitation efforts rarely serve as positive experiences for stroke and TBI patients.

> Mr. V., a 25-year-old man, incurred a TBI in a motor vehicle accident leaving him with moderate cognitive deficits and no physical disabilities. He became angry and refused to attend a vocational rehabilitation program focusing on simple reassembly tasks performed by mentally challenged adults. He eventually followed suggestions of his group and obtained a part-time job as a custodian with a private school.

Symptomatology

Groups with patients who have diverse communication disorders are also less than ideal. For example, a patient with a fluent aphasia has paraphasic speech, comprehension deficits, and prominent word-finding difficulties. The patient with nonfluent aphasia has laborious, poorly articulated speech, fair comprehension, and is noun dominant. Having these patients in the same group disrupts the flow of the session.

> Mr. C. was a 59-year-old man with severe fluent aphasia. He also had limited interests. His favorite topic of conversation was what he grew in his garden. His fluent speech allowed him to talk about this topic at every group meeting, a factor that displeased the other four patients with nonfluent aphasia in his group and often stifled discussion among them.

Similar difficulties arise when patients with severe motor speech disorders and intelligibility problems are put into groups with patients who can communicate more spontaneously.[7, 9] Often, patients with motor speech problems cannot compete verbally with more fluent patients. Their slow speech and initiation problems make interrupting them easy. In addition, the need to wait for the patient with a motor speech problem or nonfluent aphasia to communicate his or her thoughts may annoy group members who are more spontaneous in their communication efforts.

> Mr. B. was a 51-year-old man with mild Broca's aphasia and moderately severe apraxia of speech after a cerebrovascular accident (CVA). He was an active, energetic man with much to share in his group of mild aphasic men, none of whom had motor speech problems of any significance. Mr. B. became so upset with his inability to participate fully in the group's discussion that he stated he was going to quit the group. Mr. B. was moved to a group of men with similar problems and became its spokesperson.

For patients like Mr. B. and Mr. C., separate groups are advantageous. Separate groups may also be necessary when patients who rely on augmentative systems to express their needs are considered for group treatment. Similar to patients with motor speech disorders, these individuals require extra time and assistance to access and express their thoughts and feelings.

Severity

Mixed–severity level groups can also be difficult to manage. Having higher- and lower-level patients in the same group disrupts peer relationships. Mentor-student relationships can be formed among higher- and lower-level patients. Mentoring relationships can be uncomfortable for some individuals. In groups in which one high-level patient is included in a group of lower-level patients, the high-level patient may dominate to the detriment of the other patients. Conversely, one low-level patient placed within a group of higher-level patients may not have many opportunities to participate. Taking the time to allow this patient to participate may disrupt the flow of the session. Furthermore, it may annoy higher-level patients.

Rationales have been presented for treating clients with mild aphasia in group situations.[4, 7, 9, 10] These groups should be exclusive. One of the greatest benefits of group treatment is that it can disprove a patient's belief that he or she is unique and alone in his or her condition.[5, 6] For the patient with mild aphasia, this knowledge is important. Mild aphasic patients clearly understand that their problems are less severe. They may have been told how lucky they are not to have had a severe stroke.[7] The mildness of one's aphasia, however, depends on the extent to which it impairs the person's ability to communicate at the level demanded by his or her social, vocational, educational, and recreational needs.[10] These individuals can be as devastated by their handicaps as are patients with severe aphasia. Thus, they need a safe environment in which to share their concerns and to develop strategies to minimize deficits.

> Mrs. C., a 72-year-old woman with mild to moderate aphasia, was placed in a group of men with moderate to severe aphasia. She participated minimally in the group and asked the therapist if she could drop out. When asked why she stated that she felt badly about bringing up any of her problems in front of patients who were so much more severely impaired. She was placed in a high-level group and became one of its most ardent spokespersons.

Moving Mrs. C. to a homogenous group of mild aphasic patients made her much more comfortable in a group situation and helped her achieve maximum potential. Keeping her in a group of more impaired patients would have done the opposite.

Age

Experienced clinicians and clinician-managers know the problems that occur when younger patients are placed in a living situation with much older patients. Understandably, older and younger patients have different needs and interests. The former are retired, may have grown children, and are often part of a long-term marriage. Their focus is on leisure activities, health, friendships, hobbies, and other interests. Younger stroke and TBI patients, especially if they are working at the time of their injury, have different interests. Younger stroke patients, particularly those with children still at home and those who were working at the time of stroke, may have more in common with TBI patients than with older stroke patients. For most younger patients, a stroke or head injury may affect parent-child, spousal, and other relationships; cause financial difficulties; and force a change in work status.

> Mr. B. was a 45-year-old government employee with three children in college when he had a left hemisphere CVA, leaving him with Broca's aphasia and right hemiparesis. He was forced to move from a job commensurate with his college education to a clerical position at the same pay level but a lower status. This change in jobs markedly affected his self-worth and relationships within the family. He had more in common with a group composed of younger stroke and TBI patients, even though his aphasic deficits put him at a disadvantage when competing for speaking turns.

Mr. B. did well in a group of younger patients, because some of these individuals were struggling with problems similar to his (e.g., raising children, setting limits, reduced job status, sexual functioning). Older patients have fewer concerns about such problems. Because immediate patient concerns are often the focus of group work, and these concerns differ for older and younger patients, age should be considered in setting up group programs.

Gender

Gender is a less important factor in creating a homogenous group. Women have demonstrated greater anxiety and depression after a stroke than men usually experience.[11] This difference has been attributed to the fact that women tend to express their feelings more freely than men do. Women may also face the reality of their situation sooner after a stroke, because on returning home they find they are unable to resume their domestic responsibilities. Perhaps the primary reason for considering the factor of gender is that some topics (e.g., sexual functioning) may be more easily discussed in groups that are single sex.

Inclusion of Family Members

Having patients with aphasia and caregivers in the same group offers some advantages. The caregiver may learn strategies for enhancing auditory comprehension (e.g., using pauses), prompting production of specific words, and allowing extra time for processing. The benefits of such strategies include the following: (1) an improved likelihood of what the patient does in treatment generalizing to other situations; (2) additional communication opportunities for the patient; (3) better caregiver understanding of the patient's problems.

However, integrating patients and caregivers in groups has a downside. Caregivers may do all the talking, while the patients do very little. Some caregivers have problems tolerating their loved one's struggle with word retrieval and other problems. In some situations, caregivers do not speak to the aphasic members of the group, and aphasic members of the group do not use their compensatory strategies with the caregivers.[12] Alternatively, caregivers may be reluctant to discuss their concerns in the presence of persons with aphasia.

Although the clinician-manager will want to weigh carefully the pros and cons of mixing caregivers and patients, guidelines for addressing this issue are available. For example, the treatment or team leader can put some restrictions on how much talking and helping the caregiver may engage in during the session. The caregiver may observe the treatment session behind a one-way mirror rather than be present in the treatment room. If the group is one in which patients are discharged after a certain number of sessions, including the caregiver in the group sessions makes good sense, because this person might be able to provide some assistance for the patient after treatment has ended.

STANDARDS FOR PARTICIPATION

Clinicians should give careful consideration to the minimal communication, pragmatic, and behavioral standards needed by a patient to participate in a group situation. Clinicians, in concert with the supervising clinical-manager, may want to set norms for each group.[6] These norms are the implicit and explicit rules by which the group functions. If possible, they should be established early and left unchanged unless absolutely necessary.

Communication and Pragmatic Skills

Certainly, each group member needs to have sufficiently preserved pragmatic skills to know when to speak and when to keep silent. Having good listening skills and knowing how to take turns are also important. In a group, the patient with aphasia must sometimes delay attending to his or her immediate needs for the benefit of another group member with a more pressing need. The ability of a patient to form relationships with other group members may contribute to group cohesiveness. Some clinicians suggest that group cohesiveness is the analogue to the relationship of individual therapy.[1,2] This cohesiveness encompasses the patient's relationship to the group therapist, other group members, and the group as a whole.

> Mr. C., a member of a group of mild aphasic patients, attended the first portion of the group session and asked specific questions (e.g., "How can I get a new pair of glasses?"). Shortly after obtaining the answers to his questions, he excused himself and left the room. This behavior upset other group members who had questions of their own. However, Mr. C. self-terminated his involvement by moving to another city. This prompted group members to develop some rules for group admission.

Participants in groups requiring a large amount of discussion should be able to follow a conversation, remember the main topic, and contribute meaningfully to the discussion. Sometimes a patient with aphasia will demonstrate wonderful verbal skills if asked specific, personally relevant questions, but will lose track of details and be unable to become involved in a discussion. The result is sometimes reflected in off-target comments not relevant to the group's interest.

> Mr. L., a 28-year-old man, had a TBI some 12 years before joining a group for head-injury survivors. He retained a high level of verbal skills and was able to make plays on words, jokes, and so on. Mr. L., however, had a limited short-term memory and was unable to follow the thread of a discussion. When the group was engaged in an emotional discussion, Mr. L attempted to participate by turning "specific words" into jokes that were unrelated to the group discussion. In a 90-minute session, Mr. L. stopped the flow of a heated discussion 23 times with his "side" comments.

Patients like Mr. L. require a different group structure. Clinicians should recognize that some patients with aphasia will not be good group treatment members. These patients are individuals who perceive few similarities between themselves and other group members. Some patients are egocentric and refuse to share "center stage" with anyone, including the therapist. An inordinately high degree of egocentricity in one patient within a cohesive group can negatively affect group dynamics.

Social Behavior

Often a patient will possess the cognitive-communicative skills to participate in a group but display other social behaviors that disrupt the group therapy session. For example, some persons are by nature argumentative. They must win and have the last word. Others see the group meeting as a forum to lecture members of the group on their faults and have limited insight into their own problems. Argumentative, hypercritical, and highly egocentric individuals do not make good group members.

> Mr. R. was a 67-year-old man with mild anomic aphasia secondary to a stroke involving the left hemisphere. He had made an excellent recovery, and his speech and language difficulties were only noticeable to highly trained listeners. He attributed his improvement to "working hard." In group meetings he often berated others for not working hard enough and refused to acknowledge that stroke severity plays a role in improvement.

Sometimes, a patient can unknowingly interfere with the conduct of a group meeting in other socially unacceptable ways. One man I remember well came to group smelling of urine; another had alcohol on his breath. Sometimes, a group member will insist on coming to a meeting in the prodromal stages of flu or cold and risk exposing other group members. In some groups, two group members simply do not like each other. These situations require making compromises or placing the individuals in separate groups.

A common general problem in group meetings is that some patients have difficulty distinguishing topics of personal relevance to them from topics that are appropriate for group discussion. For example, the patient might bring a picture of a pet dog to share with the group. In some cases, this type of sharing might be appropriate; in others, it might not. The clinician cannot simply dismiss these good faith efforts to participate, but he or she should have an approach to limiting this type of behavior.

> Mrs. M. came to each meeting with a stack of junk mail. She had problems understanding the language of mailed credit card solicitations. She wanted to discuss each offer in the group, often insisting that the facilitator explain the contents of it to her. This bored group members and limited discussion of more important topics. This problem was resolved by limiting Mrs. M. to sharing one piece of mail per meeting.

Sometimes, aphasic stroke patients become so fixated on their own problems that they have problems operating within a group. This inward focus is apt to be observed when a patient begins a group program shortly after onset of a stroke.[11] A preoccupation with somatic and other problems may be related to the fact that much early rehabilitation is done on a one-to-one basis. The behavior manifested in the group situation is that the patient with an inward focus always wants his or her problem to be the worst.

> Mr. T., a recent stroke patient, listened as another group member, Mr. B., told of how much he missed his morning walks. Mr. T. commented that his situation was far worse. Not only could he not walk, he could not get from his easy chair to the kitchen table without having his wife help him.

Although Mr. T. has a point, many times in a group treatment session the need to talk about oneself must be sacrificed to listen to another group member.

Managing Disruptive Behaviors

When the group and the facilitator consistently spend an excessive amount of time dealing with the undesirable behavior of one member, action is warranted. Be aware of the amount of time spent in the group meeting focused on the behavior of a single individual. Have a private conference with the individual who demonstrates insensitive behaviors. Privately counsel group members in need of making behavioral changes for the good of the group, describe what these changes entail, and emphasize how positive benefits will result. If appropriate, have other group members comment on the behavior in the session and have a general discussion on the behavioral issue in the group. If these tactics fail, consider having that group member terminate participation in the group.

Although a wide range of individual behaviors can disrupt the conduct of a group meeting, the clinician cannot anticipate all possibilities. However, he or she can investigate the likelihood of a given patient having a successful group treatment experience. The clinician might speak to the patient's significant other and obtain answers to questions such as, "How do you think John would do in a group situation?" or "How well does John relate to other people?" Avoiding the inclusion of a disruptive patient in a group is better than removing the patient after he or she has started attending the group discussions.

Attendance

Once the site, time, and day of the group meeting are set, some attendance criteria are needed. As a group becomes more cohesive, regular attendance becomes important. Attendees at group meetings make more progress than nonattendees.[13] Frequent absences by a group member disrupts group harmony. Beginning each meeting with a discussion about "Where is so and so? He or she hasn't been here for 3 weeks" is awkward.

Ask group members to inform you in advance if they plan to miss a meeting. Give them a number to call or ask them to leave a message when an unanticipated illness or emergency prevents attending a meeting. Establish a policy for dismissing a patient from the group when the number of absences reaches unacceptable limits. Consider charging patients for missed meetings that are not excused.

No less important than regular attendance are the issues of tardiness and leaving early. Sometimes, these situations are not preventable. Patients may have other appointments. Traffic may have been unusually congested. In such cases, the events associated with being late or leaving early might become material for discussion within the group itself. A patient who is always late for the meeting, however, interrupts the group session as he or she enters the room, acknowledges others, and becomes situated.

Problem solve ways to improve timeliness and reduce interruptions. Counsel patients privately about the fact that being late or leaving early has a negative impact on the group's function. Many other sources of interruption can be found in group meetings. I have never had a member bring a cellular telephone to a meeting, but beepers (or pagers) have gone off. However, the most frequent source of interruption is when a patient needs to leave the meeting to use the bathroom. This type of interruption is preventable with a simple reminder to patients to use the facilities before the meeting starts.

ADMISSIONS, DISCHARGES, AND NEW MEMBERS

The clinician responsible for running the group and keeping it organized should have some guidelines for admission, discharge, and accepting new members.

Admissions

Group treatment literature does not reveal a specific time for starting group treatment. Aphasic stroke patients may become involved in a group relatively soon after a stroke, after a period of individual treatment, or when aphasia has become chronic. The timing is less important than the selection of group treatment as the best method for treating a particular patient. Some patients with aphasia may express reluctance to join a group. A helpful technique is to have the patient meet a few group members and attend a few sessions before making a final decision on participation. The clinician can facilitate a patient's transition into a group by highlighting the benefits of group treatment earlier rather than later. In no case should having a patient participate in a group be presented as something less than optimal. Group treatment should not be cast as a "poor second" to individual treatment.

Discharges

In some cases, patients attend group therapy as long as they meet the standards of group behavior and attendance.[4] Other groups have limits on how long a patient can attend group therapy.[3] Transitional groups that provide support for stroke patients moving from one rehabilitation setting to another admit and discharge patients regularly.[8, 11] When a patient is discharged from group treatment, preparing the patient and fellow group members for this event is important. Some group members become alarmed when they suddenly realize that Mr. B. is no longer present. Tell them in advance that Mr. B. will be leaving the group or "graduating" on a certain date. If a patient decides to self-terminate group therapy, ask him or her to inform the other group members of this decision rather than to stop attending without notice. Group members develop bonds and mutual respect for one another. Keeping fellow group members informed about a decision to drop out of the group is the respectable thing to do.

New Members

Develop a policy for bringing new patients into the group. Determine whether new admissions are to be the clinician's decision alone or whether group members have a voice. In one of my mild aphasia groups, patients were accepted on a trial basis.[14] Group members were forewarned that a new person was coming to the group and that they had a say in determining whether the new person should join the group. No one was ever refused membership, but I believe that asking members for their opinion was important. Another possibility is to have a new group member commit to attending a minimum of three group sessions and then make a decision regarding further involvement.

LEADERSHIP

The leadership of the group is important to its success.[15] Because all groups have different purposes and compositions, no criteria for the perfect leader exist. Whatever title is accorded this person (e.g., leader, facilitator, director, therapist), he or she should be a seasoned clinician, well-trained in counseling. I have a strong personal bias that this person should be a professional. Without significant guidance from a professional, well-intended stroke survivors and laypersons seldom have the training, experience, knowledge, and broad-based perspective necessary to manage a group of persons with aphasia.

Leadership Characteristics

Yalom, in a book that should be considered a Bible of group therapy, identifies some group leadership functions that relate to outcomes.[5] These functions include (1) the ability to provide emotional stimulation through the use of confrontation, modeling, encouraging risk-taking, and self-disclosure; (2) caring, through the offering of support, affection, warmth, concern, and genuineness; (3) meaning attribution, accomplished by exploring, interpreting, and clarifying, and by providing a cognitive framework for change; and (4) executive function, achieved by setting limits, establishing rules, managing time, and suggesting procedures.

Most group members respond more positively to a democratic climate than to an authoritarian one.[15] A warm, accepting, democratic style is used by most good group leaders, but individual differences occur among leaders. Some writers have attempted to create characteristic leadership styles based on studies and observation.[16] For example, "warmies" are accepting and patient leaders. They are slow to judge behavior and hesitant to set goals and directives. "Pushers" function at a high energy level. They confront, using humor or criticism, and are quick to mix, fight, and take chances. "Bad leaders" are defensive and out of touch with their own feelings and needs. They have little understanding of the group process. Sensitive and productive leaders appropriately combine warm and pushy characteristics to obtain the necessary results.

For a group to succeed, the leader must value what he or she is doing, sense that individual and group goals are being met, and commit to the process. The improvement course after a brain injury is a long journey, and the patient's ability to cope with the residuals of the brain injury is different at 1 month, 1 year, and 2 years postictus.[17] Different leadership styles are needed in accordance with the group composition and goals.

Coleadership

Certain groups may benefit from coleadership. Members of the health care team who might combine in various ways to colead a group are the speech-language pathologist, social worker, psychologist, psychiatrist, occupational therapist, and recreational therapist.[11, 13, 18, 19] Some of the programs presented in the synopsis on group treatment approaches in Chapters 5 and 6 reflect the use of coleadership.

The title accorded the person responsible for the group is largely determined by that person's role in the group. *Leaders* take a more direct role in organizing group activities by asking questions, ensuring that all group members are participating in the session, initiating discussion topics, preparing and supplying materials, and providing feedback. *Facilitators* have an indirect role in group treatment. Their job is to offer guidance when needed and intervene only when requested by group members. They keep the discussion on track, clarify statements, attitudes, and feelings. Both leaders and facilitators must work together to ensure continuity of discussion topic issues from one group session to the next.

Experience

If you are a clinician-manager starting a group program, determine whether staff members with sufficient experience are available to conduct a group. If existing staff lack these skills, perhaps the new group can be started in collaboration with another clinician (e.g., neuropsychologist, clinical social worker, or physician) who has experience in group treatment work. Group treatment programs may already exist in your facility. In such instances, consider observing some of the sessions.

REFERENCES

1. Pachalska M. Group therapy for aphasia patients. Aphasiology 1991;5:541.
2. Fawcus M. Group Therapy: A Learning Situation. In C Code, D Muller (eds), Aphasia Therapy. London: Edward Arnold, 1983;113.
3. Avent J. Manual of Cooperative Group Treatment for Aphasia. Boston: Butterworth–Heinemann, 1997;1.
4. Marshall RC. Problem-focused group treatment for clients with mild aphasia. Am J Speech-Lang Pathol 1993;3:31.
5. Yalom ID. The Theory and Practice of Group Psychotherapy (3rd ed). New York: Basic Books, 1985;3.
6. Luterman DM. Counseling Persons with Communicative Disorders and Their Families (3rd ed). Austin, TX: Pro-Ed, 1996;111.
7. Marshall RC. Problem-Solving Support Groups for Long-Term Brain Injured Adults. Paper presented at the American Speech-Language-Hearing Association Convention, Boston, November 1997.
8. Singler JK. The Stroke Group. In M Seligman (ed), Group Psychotherapy and Counseling with Special Populations. Baltimore: University Park, 1977;43.
9. Marshall RC. A Problem-Focused Group Program for Clients with Mild Aphasia. In R Elman (ed), Group Treatment of Aphasia: The Expert Clinician's Approach. Boston: Butterworth–Heinemann, 1999.
10. Linebaugh C. Mild Aphasia. In A Holland (ed), Language Disorders in Adults. San Diego: College Hill, 1984;113.
11. Bucher J, Smith E, Gillespie C. Short-term group therapy for stroke patients in a rehabilitation centre. Br J Med Psychol 1984;57:283.
12. Fox L, Fried-Oken, M. Trial Implementation of Communicative Autonomy Treatment in a Group Environment. Unpublished manuscript. Eugene, OR: University of Oregon, 1996.
13. Rice B, Paul A, Muller DJ. An evaluation of a social support group for spouses of aphasic partners. Aphasiology 1987;1:247.
14. Aten J, Kushner-Vogel D, Haire A, Fitch-West J. Group Treatment for Aphasia: A Panel Discussion. In R Brookshire (ed), Clinical Aphasiology Conference Proceedings. Minneapolis: BRK, 1981;141.
15. Seligman M. Group Psychotherapy and Counseling with Special Populations. Baltimore: University Park, 1977;1

16. Bebout J. Warmth and Pushiness in Group Leaders. The Group Leader's Workbook. New York: Explorations Institute, 1972;1.
17. Lyon J. Coping with Aphasia. San Diego: Singular, 1998;1.
18. Fox L. Recreation-Focused Treatment and Generalization of Language Skills in Aphasic Patients. Paper presented at the American Speech-Language-Hearing Association Convention, Seattle, November 1990.
19. Goldwasser AN, Auerbach SM, Harkins SW. Cognitive, affective, and behavioral effects of reminiscence group therapy on demented elderly. Int J Aging Hum Dev 1987;25:209.

II

Treatment Methods

6

Prerequisites to Group Treatment

Group treatment is different from individual treatment. In most cases, patients with aphasia start group treatment after undergoing individual treatment. Group treatment sessions also occur less frequently than individual sessions. Most groups have different compositions and multiple purposes.[1, 2] For example, in higher-level groups, participants may work on improving spoken narrative performance or verbal problem solving. In lower-level groups, the use of total communication, compensatory techniques, and other strategies to enhance message transmission in whatever way possible may be stressed. Group treatment is often interactive and somewhat holistic and therefore differs from the modality-based (e.g., auditory comprehension training) and stimulus-response (e.g., sentence completion tasks) of individual treatment. In those groups with a strong psychosocial focus (e.g., overcoming communication barriers, developing self-confidence, and discussion of mutual problems related to stroke), communication may only be addressed indirectly.

EXPECTATIONS

Because group treatment is different, clinicians and patients should think about their expectations. These expectations may need to be altered for some patients. For example, an aphasic patient without funds to pay for individual treatment might be placed in a small group in the early postonset period. The patient may improve, but this improvement may not equal or occur as rapidly in the group situation as might have occurred in individual treatment.

Most patients do not begin group treatment until the aphasia is chronic. Less improvement is expected for these patients because treatment is not aided by the boost of spontaneous recovery. In addition, within the group situation the clinician divides his or her time among several persons rather than devoting it to a single individual. Group patients have fewer turns and opportunities for practice than do patients who are treated individually. In general, expecting patients to progress as rapidly in group situations as in individual treatment is not reasonable. The results of the Veterans Administration (VA) cooperative study previously described in Chapter 4 suggest that this is not always the case. Remember that patients entered the VA study at 4 weeks postonset and had not had prior individual treatment.

PREREQUISITE BACKGROUND INFORMATION ON GROUP PATIENTS

An axiom for students in my aphasia class is that good aphasia clinicians know their patients and their families. This type of relationship with patients is vital if we are to show how group treatment helps. For example, to illustrate improvements in communicative status resulting from group treatment, the clinician should know something about the patient's communication status before the stroke and before beginning group treatment. To attribute psychosocial improvements (e.g., participating in formerly enjoyed activities) to group treatment, the clinician should know what the patient's interests, activities, and participation levels were before the stroke.

Consider the patient who stops going to church after a stroke because he is embarrassed by his uncontrolled crying (i.e., emotional lability). If group discussions center on understanding and controlling emotional behavior and the patient resumes attending Sunday services, group therapy may have had something to do with this behavior change. Unless the clinician knows something about the patient's premorbid lifestyle, this important information will be missed. Some strategies for obtaining the required background information are discussed here.

Biography

An easy way to learn about the patient with aphasia is to have a significant other (SO) write a biography about the patient. Tell the SO that the information will help you know the patient better and aid in planning treatment. Also, make sure the SO does not become caught up in the mechanics of writing the document. Instead, he or she should focus on information about the patient's education, friends, hobbies and interests, likes and dislikes, significant life experiences, and work history. Assure the SO that whatever he or she provides will help as long as you can read it.

Supplement the biographical information with photographs, newspaper clippings, and other items of importance in the patient's life. If appropriate, ask the patient and SO to provide a few statements that address their hopes for the future. Family members are usually very willing to create a personal portfolio for the person with aphasia. Typically, they see this task as a way of participating in the treatment process.

Informational Questionnaire

Developing an informational questionnaire to obtain background information on patients and family members may be helpful. Items in the questionnaire can be tailored to meet the demands of your work situation. Appendix 6.1 contains a list of questions that when answered by a caregiver or SO might provide useful background information on the patient entering group treatment. The questionnaire uses the term "spouse," but any individual who knows the patient well can complete this form. The questionnaire should be completed before the patient starts group treatment. You can use subsets of questions to create a document that is appropriate for the work setting.

The questionnaire can be administered before the patient enters group treatment and readministered at a later point in time. When the questionnaire is administered again later in group treatment, it provides some objective evidence of changes in the patient's activity pattern during group treatment. Items contained in this questionnaire not only provide background information about the stroke patient with aphasia but about the caregiver as well. This information will give the clinician an idea of the distribution of responsibilities in the household and how these responsibilities may have been redistributed after the stroke.

Communication History

No less important than obtaining relevant patient and family background information is finding out as much as possible about the patient's premorbid communicative status, patterns, and habits. Green provides a set of interview questions for exploring premorbid communication interests and habits of persons with aphasia.[4] Her interview covers several specific topic areas: language used, possible speech problems, communication style, types of communication, timing of communications, persons spoken to, communication topics, communication environments, comprehension, reading, writing, and gesturing skills. Table 6.1 presents Green's interview questions.

Swindell et al. have also developed a questionnaire for surveying the personal and communicative style of persons with aphasia.[5] Respondents rate personal style characteristics (e.g., perfectionism) on a 5-point

Table 6.1
Topics on preaphasia communication questionnaire.

---

1. Language used: How many languages did the person speak/understand/read/write? What were they? Where was the language used?
2. Speech: Did the person have any speech problems before the stroke? Describe. What did the person do when stuck for a word?
3. Style: Was the person talkative/quiet/argumentative/responsive to social chatter/a fast talker/a good listener/dogmatic/thoughtful/dominant/hesitant/passive/ understandable/forgetful of names/a bad listener?
4. Type: Did the person answer the telephone/telephone people/answer the door/talk in shops, bars, buses, banks, cars, churches, at meals/play board or card games/give public talks/do interviews/pray aloud/sing/ attend meetings? Who usually started conversations? Who led conversations? Who finished conversations?
5. Timing: When did the person do most of his/her talking? Set time (e.g., at breakfast, after work)? When did he/she seldom talk? When did he/she talk most to you?
6. People: Whom does the person talk to (e.g., neighbors, spouse, family, friends, coworkers, strangers)? Whom does he/she talk to most often? Did he/she ever talk to groups of people (specify size, type of people, topics, situation)?
7. Topics: What does the person like to talk about (e.g., news, television, politics, religion)? What specific viewpoints did he/she have? What topics were avoided? What kinds of things did you talk to him/her about?
8. Environment: What kind of environments did the person talk in (e.g., noisy/quiet, public/private, small/large, inside/outside)? Where did he/she do most of his/her talking (e.g., work, home)?
9. Comprehension: Did the person watch television, listen to the radio, listen to lectures or sermons, go to the movies, or go to the theater?
10. Reading: Did the person read? What (letters, magazines, books, newspapers, technical articles)? How often? Did he/she read aloud?
11. Writing: Did the person write? What (letters, shopping lists, postcards, forms, stories)? How often? To whom? About what?
12. Gesturing: How did the person use his/her hands or face when talking?

Source: Reprinted with permission from G Green. Communication in aphasia therapy: some of the procedures and issues involved. Br J Dis Commun 1984;19:35.

scale and respond affirmatively or negatively to communication style questions (e.g., he or she is artistic). The authors point out that information from this questionnaire may be useful in planning treatment, setting treatment goals, and personalizing treatment. Although not developed for use in aphasia groups, information from the questionnaire would seem to be helpful data to collect on patients entering group treatment. See Figure 6.1 for an example of this questionnaire.

I. Personal style

For each of the following statements circle the number from 1 to 5 that best fits your family member.

A. Perfectionist	1	2	3	4	5	Tolerant of imperfection
B. Easily influenced	1	2	3	4	5	Tends to take charge
C. Sees one solution to problem	1	2	3	4	5	Sees many ways to solve a problem
D. Dependent	1	2	3	4	5	Independent
E. Keeps to self	1	2	3	4	5	Outgoing
F. Does not show much humor	1	2	3	4	5	Has a good sense of humor
G. Lacks confidence	1	2	3	4	5	Confident
H. Too self-critical	1	2	3	4	5	Appropriately self-critical
I. Expects the worst	1	2	3	4	5	Expects the best
J. Overwhelmed by problems	1	2	3	4	5	Challenged and stimulated by problems
K. Does not know self well	1	2	3	4	5	Knows self well
L. Rigid	1	2	3	4	5	Flexible
M. Stays down when things go wrong	1	2	3	4	5	Bounces back easily
N. Easily thrown off-balance	1	2	3	4	5	Takes things in stride
O. Thinks things will work out badly	1	2	3	4	5	Thinks things will turn out OK

II. Communicative style

Read the statements below. Decide if the statement describes your family member. If it does, write a plus (+) sign after the statement. If it does not, write a minus (−) sign.
1. When giving directions, would be more likely to draw a map than to tell the directions.
2. When doodling, tends to make figures (e.g., people) and geometric forms rather than words.
3. Paints and draws as part of work or hobby.
4. Can usually tell how others feel by their facial expressions.
5. Talks with hands.
6. Is an artistic or creative person.
7. Uses demonstrating gestures to help explain something.
8. Maintains correspondence with at least one other person.
9. More likely to complain by writing a letter than making a phone call.
10. Regularly makes lists (e.g., things to do).
11. Leaves notes for other people.
12. Job involves a lot of paperwork.
13. When sending greeting cards, tends to include a message beyond the signature.
14. Keeps and uses appointment book.
15. Depends on newspapers and magazines to keep up with current events.
16. Makes use of references such as dictionaries and phone books.
17. Tends to read instructions for something first rather than "jumping in."
18. Reads the equivalent of a book a month or more.

Figure 6.1 Questionnaire to evaluate personal and communicative style.

19. Job involves a lot of reading.
20. Subscribes to magazines or newspaper or book clubs.
21. Takes what he/she reads seriously.
22. Really likes to talk.
23. Tends to express anger in words rather than "walking out" or "clamming up."
24. Is a good joke or story teller.
25. Has a way with words.
26. Is good at imitating different accents.
27. Is the "life of the party."
28. Work involves a lot of speaking.
29. Is a good listener.
30. Job requires a lot of listening to others.
31. Rarely interrupts others when they are talking.
32. Usually waits for answer to a question that he/she asks.
33. Is usually interested in what other people have to say.
34. Enjoys listening to lectures and sermons.
35. Prefers to hear about others rather than talk about self.

Figure 6.1 Continued

REFERENCES

1. Kearns KP. Group Therapy for Aphasia: Theoretical and Practical Considerations. In R Chapey (ed), Language Intervention Strategies in Adult Aphasia (3rd ed). Baltimore: Williams & Wilkins, 1994;304.
2. Kearns KP, Simmons NN. Group Therapy for Aphasia: A Survey of Veterans Administration Medical Centers. In RH Brookshire (ed), Clinical Aphasiology Conference Proceedings. Minneapolis: BRK, 1985;176.
3. Wertz RT, Collins MH, Weiss D, et al. Veterans Administration cooperative study on aphasia. A comparison of individual and group treatment. J Speech Hear Res 1981;24:580.
4. Green G. Communication in aphasia therapy: some of the procedures and issues involved. Br J Disord Commun 1984;19:35.
5. Swindell C, Pashek G, Holland A. A Questionnaire for Surveying Personal and Communicative Style. In RH Brookshire (ed), Clinical Aphasiology Conference Proceedings. Minneapolis: BRK, 1982;50.

Appendix 6.1

Questionnaire Items

	Strongly Agree						Strongly Disagree

1. My spouse needs assistance from me dressing him-/herself. SA |‒‒|‒‒|‒‒|‒‒|‒‒| SD

2. My spouse needs assistance from me caring for him-/herself. SA |‒‒|‒‒|‒‒|‒‒|‒‒| SD

3. Since the stroke, my spouse does not use the telephone as much as before. SA |‒‒|‒‒|‒‒|‒‒|‒‒| SD

4. My spouse is unable to adjust the tuning on the television. SA |‒‒|‒‒|‒‒|‒‒|‒‒| SD

5. My spouse is capable of taking part in community activities. SA |‒‒|‒‒|‒‒|‒‒|‒‒| SD

6. My spouse was socially outgoing before the stroke. SA |‒‒|‒‒|‒‒|‒‒|‒‒| SD

7. My spouse expects me to be with him/her all the time. SA |‒‒|‒‒|‒‒|‒‒|‒‒| SD

8. My spouse is able to make simple decisions (e.g., what to wear). SA |‒‒|‒‒|‒‒|‒‒|‒‒| SD

9. My spouse would rather not entertain at all.

SA __|__|__|__|__|__|__ SD

10. Now, my spouse cannot manage money for the household.

SA __|__|__|__|__|__|__ SD

11. My spouse prefers to sit rather than do things.

SA __|__|__|__|__|__|__ SD

12. Before the stroke, my spouse enjoyed talking very much.

SA __|__|__|__|__|__|__ SD

13. My spouse needs help with feeding him-/herself.

SA __|__|__|__|__|__|__ SD

14. When we are with others, my spouse expects me to interpret what he/she is trying to say.

SA __|__|__|__|__|__|__ SD

15. Since the stroke, my spouse tries to be as active socially as he/she can.

SA __|__|__|__|__|__|__ SD

16. At times, my spouse acts like a child.

SA __|__|__|__|__|__|__ SD

17. Before the stroke, my spouse was always on the telephone.

SA __|__|__|__|__|__|__ SD

18. My spouse would rather entertain smaller groups of people than larger groups of people.

SA __|__|__|__|__|__|__ SD

19. My spouse likes to have assistance from

me caring for
him-/herself.   SA |___|___|___|___|___|___| SD

20. My spouse would
rather write things
down than tell me.   SA |___|___|___|___|___|___| SD

21. My spouse enjoys
going to parties and
other affairs.   SA |___|___|___|___|___|___| SD

22. My spouse needs to
have me attending
to him/her at all
times.   SA |___|___|___|___|___|___| SD

23. My spouse enjoys
going to town.   SA |___|___|___|___|___|___| SD

24. My spouse does not
enjoy entertaining as
much as he/she did
before the stroke.   SA |___|___|___|___|___|___| SD

25. Before the stroke,
my spouse managed
the money for our
house.   SA |___|___|___|___|___|___| SD

26. Before the stroke,
my spouse was very
demanding of my
time.   SA |___|___|___|___|___|___| SD

27. At present, my
spouse avoids
talking with people.   SA |___|___|___|___|___|___| SD

28. My spouse thinks
that he/she cannot
do anything.   SA |___|___|___|___|___|___| SD

29. My spouse does
not voluntarily
associate with others.   SA |___|___|___|___|___|___| SD

30. My spouse would rather watch television than visit the neighbors.

SA ⎿__I___I___I___I___I___I__⏌ SD

31. My spouse likes to have help from me feeding him-/herself.

SA ⎿__I___I___I___I___I___I__⏌ SD

32. Now my spouse is very demanding of me and my time.

SA ⎿__I___I___I___I___I___I__⏌ SD

33. My spouse avoids social activities whenever he/she can.

SA ⎿__I___I___I___I___I___I__⏌ SD

34. My spouse does not use our checking or savings account now.

SA ⎿__I___I___I___I___I___I__⏌ SD

35. The only friends my spouse has are other stroke victims.

SA ⎿__I___I___I___I___I___I__⏌ SD

36. Before the stroke, my spouse did not enjoy taking vacations.

SA ⎿__I___I___I___I___I___I__⏌ SD

37. My spouse likes to have help from me with dressing.

SA ⎿__I___I___I___I___I___I__⏌ SD

38. My spouse needs help in selecting the television show he/she wants to watch.

SA ⎿__I___I___I___I___I___I__⏌ SD

39. The only activity my spouse has is to watch television.

SA ⎿__I___I___I___I___I___I__⏌ SD

40. My spouse looks forward to our vacations.

SA ⎿__I___I___I___I___I___I__⏌ SD

7

Synopsis of Group Treatment Programs for Aphasia

A 1994 comprehensive literature review on group treatment of patients with aphasia identified three primary treatment approaches: psychosocial, family counseling and support, and speech and language.[1] The speech and language menu encompassed (1) direct language treatment, (2) indirect language treatment, (3) sociolinguistic treatment, (4) transition, and (5) maintenance groups. A survey of group treatment programs for aphasia in Department of Veterans Administration medical centers revealed that most aphasia groups have multiple goals and that strict classification of aphasia treatment groups as one type or another is difficult.[2]

This synopsis of group treatment focuses on two broad program types: those with a communication focus and those with a psychosocial focus. The former are usually directed by speech-language pathologists. Outcomes are expressed as changes in measures of speech and language target behaviors and pragmatic indicators. Psychosocial-focused programs are often cofacilitated. The goals of such programs are to enhance participation in life (e.g., leisure, work, and games) and improve coping skills of aphasic stroke patients and their families. Outcomes are expressed with measures of well-being and other scales. In this chapter, I also provide limited information on transition groups. The objective of groups is to assist recent stroke victims, some who may be aphasic, accept, adjust to, and cope with the physical, communicative, and cognitive residuals of stroke. A need for such groups may develop as a stroke victim moves from an acute care setting to a rehabilitation site, or from a rehabilitation setting to an outpatient setting. Group treatment is facilitated by a range of professionals (e.g., physician, social worker, psychiatrist, nurse). Outcome measures are usually not provided for these groups.

Because this synopsis presents information on aphasia groups in three basic sections—communication, psychosocial, and transitional—

two caveats are necessary. First, substantial overlap exists among all group treatment endeavors. Second, this synopsis is not all-inclusive. In selecting those programs to be included in the synopsis, my bias was to include more of those programs that were data-based programs. I define *data-based* simply as those in which those responsible for the program attempted to quantify the effects of treatment.

To facilitate comparison of the group programs presented, the following organizational schema was adopted:

1. Information on group composition (e.g., What was severity and type of aphasia? prerequisite verbal skills? etiology?)
2. Time postonset (e.g., When did patients begin the group program?)
3. Amount of treatment (e.g., What was the frequency and duration of treatment? length of treatment sessions?)
4. Objectives (e.g., What were the general treatment goals for the group?)
5. Representative activities (e.g., What is an example of a treatment activity carried out in the group situation?)
6. Results (e.g., What was measured to show that participants improved as a result of group treatment?)
7. Special features (e.g., What, if any, features distinguish this group program from other programs?)

COMMUNICATION-FOCUSED GROUPS

Most group treatment programs in which the overall goal is to improve the patient's communication attempt to group patients according to severity of their aphasia. In addition, group therapy for most patients begins when the aphasia is chronic or after individual treatment has ended. Frequency and duration of treatment and number of persons included in each group varies for the studies reviewed. Most of the programs reviewed measure changes in communication status in one of three ways: traditional speech and language measures, functional measures, or with communication rating scales.

Veterans Administration Cooperative Study on Aphasia[3]

Composition: Patients with aphasia falling between the fifteenth and seventy-fifth overall percentile on the Porch Index of Communicative Ability (PICA).[4] Participants also met other rigid selection criteria.
Time postonset: All patients began treatment at 4 weeks postonset.
Amount of treatment: Groups of three to seven patients received 4 hours of group treatment from a therapist per week. Group treat-

ment was supplemented by 4 hours of recreational activities per week. Duration of treatment was 44 weeks.

Objectives: Facilitation of language use in a social setting. Direct manipulation of speech or language deficits was not used.

Representative activities: Discussing current events, attending lectures, watching movies with controversial themes, taking field trips, singing with groups, and engaging in mutual problem solving (e.g., helping an aphasic patient decide whether to marry and, if so, who to marry).[5]

Results: Patients were evaluated every 11 weeks with a battery of language measures. Significant gains were reported on modality and overall means for the PICA. See Chapters 2 and 4 for additional information on the results of this study.

Special features: This study is the only one in which patients who received group treatment did not receive individual treatment first.

Group Treatment in Aphasia Using Cooperative Learning Methods[6]

Composition: Eight patients with aphasia whose Western Aphasia Battery (WAB)[7] aphasia quotients (AQs) were between 58 and 97. Patients with equivalent AQs were seen in two-person groups.

Time postonset: All patients were at least 1 year postonset.

Amount of treatment: Groups met for approximately 18 sessions of 45–90 minutes.

Objectives: To improve narrative and procedural discourse and overall language performance through the use of cooperative learning principles.[6, 8] These learning principles include (1) positive independence (working together to complete tasks in treatment); (2) face-to-face primitive interaction (assisting, supporting, and encouraging the learning from each other); (3) individual accountability and responsibility (receiving feedback about performance and discussing how to improve performance); (4) using collaborative skills (decision making, trust building, communication, and dealing with conflicts); and (5) group processing (discussion of progress toward goals and maintaining effective working relationships).

Representative activities: Treatment materials included narrative and procedural stories that varied in length and complexity based on patient severity levels. The two aphasic patients alternate between assuming roles of recaller and facilitator. The recaller retells the target story. The facilitator corrects, prompts, and adds missing information as needed. More specific information on this method is provided in Chapter 8.

Results: Cooperative group learning methods markedly improved the content (measured by number of content-information units) of narrative and procedural discourse for three of eight patients. Patients who improved showed generalization of their performance to untrained narrative and procedural discourse tasks.

Special features: In this treatment approach, the clinician does not lead but creates a cooperative learning environment by providing an atmosphere of support and guidance that encourages aphasic patients to help each other. He or she creates the environment by structuring the session, supplying the stories, collecting data, and teaching the patients cueing strategies.

Group Communication Intervention with Chronically Aphasic Persons[9]

Composition: Patients representing a variety of aphasia classifications with overall PICA scores ranging from the twenty-fifth to seventy-sixth percentiles. Treatment groups were formed on the basis of patient scores on the Communicative Activities of Daily Living (CADL).[10] Patients with CADL scores (136 possible) below 105 formed a low group; those with scores above 120 formed a high group.

Time postonset: The amount of time ranged from 20 to 155 months.

Amount of treatment: Patients were seen in groups for 1 hour three times per week for 20 weeks. This phase was followed by a 10-week no-treatment period, an added 20 weeks of treatment, and a second 10-week no-treatment period.

Objectives: (1) To determine whether functional communication therapy (FCT) produces changes in a chronic aphasic patient's performance on a standardized test (PICA); (2) to determine whether FCT produces changes in a test measuring functional communication (CADL); and (3) to determine whether any improvement following FCT treatment is maintained after treatment is withdrawn.

Representative activities: Two forms of treatment were used in the study. Contemporary group treatment (CTG) involved greetings and socialization (e.g., discussion of personal and current events), core activities (e.g., cooking), sharing of life experiences using an established vocabulary, sequencing of activities, use of key words, and specific communication activities (e.g., repetition, category naming). Structured television viewing group treatment (STVGT) helped patients develop strategies to enhance comprehension and expression of communication intents of television programs.

Results: Group means on both the CADL and PICA overall were significantly higher after the initial 20-week treatment. Gains on these measures were maintained after the first no-treatment period. Both groups improved on the PICA but not the CADL after the second 20-

week treatment period. Gains on the PICA, but not on the CADL, were maintained after the second no-treatment period.

Special features: STVGT and CTG treatments were systematically alternated for 10-week periods during the two 20-week treatment intervals.

Group Therapy to Encourage Communication Ability in Aphasic Patients[11]

Composition: This was an open-ended group for all patients who recovered from stroke and had aphasia. No other information about severity or type of aphasia is provided.

Time postonset: When patients begin group treatment cannot be determined from the information provided. The authors report that their institution is the only treatment center for aphasia in Slovenia. The impression is that group treatment may be started early with aphasic patients in this country.

Amount of treatment: Groups of four to seven patients (maximum is 10) meet twice per week for 1 hour.

Objectives: (1) Decrease emotional tension; (2) prevent social isolation; (3) encourage the need for communication; (4) encourage the ability to search for, develop, and use communication in social situations; and (5) develop confidence and self-respect.

Representative activities: Stages of communication through which the group is moved by the therapists include (1) feeling and perceiving the closeness of others; (2) recognizing the messages of others; (3) reacting to messages of others; and (4) communicating with others and sharing experiences with others.

Results: A five-point scale of communication was used to assess the effects of treatment. Pre- and post-treatment ratings on the scale of communication for 108 patients reflect improvement for most patients. Patients who attended at least 10 sessions were found to improve most.

Group Communication Treatment for Individuals with Chronic Aphasia[12]

Composition: Twenty-eight patients with aphasia secondary to a left hemisphere cerebrovascular accident (CVA) with overall percentile rankings on the shortened PICA (SPICA)[13] between the tenth and ninetieth percentiles.

Time postonset: Patients were at least 6 months postonset and had completed all individual therapy available to them. Patients also met other selection criteria: 80 years of age or younger, no major medical complications, premorbid literacy in English, and signed informed consent.

Amount of treatment: The 28 patients were randomly assigned to subject pools. Pool 1 subjects received immediate assessment and structured group communication treatment by a speech-language pathologist. This consisted of two 3-hour treatment periods per week for 4 months. Two separate groups of seven patients were created for mild and moderate aphasic subjects. Pool 2 subjects received immediate assessment but deferred communication treatment. In the deferred period they attended weekly performance, support, social, or movement groups in which they could socialize, but they did not participate in structured group activities. Separate groups of seven patients were established for subjects with mild and moderate aphasia.

Objectives: This study was designed to answer two questions: (1) Does group communication treatment result in changes on linguistic measures such as the SPICA and WAB? (2) Will group communication treatment result in change on a functional measure such as the CADL?

Representative activities: (1) Improving patient's ability to convey a message using his or her most useful strategy; (2) increasing initiation in conversational exchanges; (3) expanding self-awareness of personal goals and recognition of progress; and (4) promoting confidence in personally relevant communication situations.

Research findings: A repeated measures analysis of variance collapsing results for mild and moderately impaired subjects was used to compare changes for subjects in Pool 1 and Pool 2 across the 4-month treatment period. Subjects who received structured group treatment made statistically significant gains on the SPICA, WAB, and CADL. Pool 2 subjects, deferred treatment, did not make significant changes on any of the dependent measures.

Special features: This study, being prepared for publication at the time of this writing, is the only one of its kind in which the effects of group treatment are examined in relation to a nontreated group.

Functional Communication Therapy for Chronic Aphasic Patients[14]

Composition: Seven patients with Broca's aphasia. Patients had pretreatment overall percentile scores on the PICA ranging from the thirtieth to the seventy-third percentiles.

Time postonset: This period ranged from 9 to 262 months (mean, 97.9 months).

Objective: To improve functional communication in selected communicative situations.

Amount of treatment: Patients were seen twice weekly in 1-hour sessions over a 12-week period.

Representative activities: Role-playing to elicit relevant responses in the following situations: (1) shopping in a grocery and variety store; (2) giving and following directions; (3) engaging in social greetings and exchanges; (4) supplying personal information; (5) reading signs and directories; and (6) using gestures to express ideas. Each week was focused on a different topic for the first 6 weeks. The second 6-week treatment period replicated the first.

Results: Patients showed no change in pre- and post-treatment PICA overall scores. Pre- to post-treatment changes on the CADL were higher for all patients, and significantly higher for the group after therapy. Administration of the CADL 6 weeks after cessation of treatment revealed that these changes had been maintained.

Problem-Focused Group Treatment for Clients with Mild Aphasia[15]

Composition: Twenty-five patients with mild aphasia; overall scores on the PICA ranged from the sixty-first to ninetieth percentiles.

Time postonset: Patients entered the group between 2 and 400 months postonset (mean, 37 months).

Amount of treatment: Six to 10 patients met once per week for 1 hour. Group members are allowed to participate in these sessions as long as they like.

Objectives: Reduce the psychosocial effects of aphasia; improve the social, vocational, and recreational integration; provide a safe environment to discuss physical, psychological, and social consequences of brain injury; provide sufficient space to develop initiative.

Representative activities: Group members are responsible for identifying specific everyday problems related to communication and cognition. Solutions to the problems are worked out collaboratively in the group. For example, meeting a new person after a stroke was a problem for some group members. In response to one aphasic patient's avowed fear of dating because of embarrassing word-finding problems, the group suggested that he put a personal ad in the local paper. The details of the ad, the responses to the ad, and the patient's responses to the responders were discussed in the group.

Results: Fourteen of 18 patients who regularly attended group meetings for more than 1 year showed improvements on overall, gestural, verbal, and graphic scores for the PICA.

Cooperative Group Treatment for Individuals with Mild Aphasia[16]

Composition: Two patients with anomic aphasia as determined by the WAB.[7] Patients had mild comprehension deficits, anomia in connected speech, and paragraph level reading and writing skills; shared common interests; and were highly motivated.

Time postonset: One patient began the treatment program at 1 year postonset. This information is not provided for the second patient.

Amount of treatment: Two 1-hour biweekly treatment sessions over a 2-month period (18 sessions total). The first four sessions were devoted to assessment with the WAB, Boston Naming Test,[17] and American Speech-Language-Hearing Association Functional Assessment of Communication Skills[18] as well as administration of probes to establish baseline levels of performance on narrative and procedural discourse tasks (e.g., retelling stories). The last 14 sessions were devoted to treatment of narrative and procedural discourse.

Objectives: Quantifiable goals included (1) improving the content of narrative and procedural discourse and (2) increasing cueing skills when acting as the facilitator during the treatment session. Qualitative goals were to (1) increase dependency on each other and to decrease dependency on the clinician, (2) increase awareness of improvement in communication skills, and (3) increase self-confidence as communicators.

Representative activities: (1) Clinician reads target story (e.g., a narrative about Hawaii). (2) Patients work together to create a list of 10 key words or phrases about the story (e.g., Oahu, blue sky) and record the elements on a sheet. (3) In the cued recall stage, the patient selected as the recaller practices retelling the story. When he or she hits a snag or has a word-finding problem, the other patient (the facilitator) provides cues until all key words or phrases are recalled. (4) In the recall probe stage, the recaller is to retell the story in 1 minute without assistance. (5) In a brief feedback stage, the facilitator provides feedback to the recaller, and the recaller provides feedback to the facilitator about the effectiveness of the cueing. The clinician provides feedback to both.

Research findings: One patient showed a marked increase in generalization probe scores from pre- to post-treatment.

Recreation-Focused Treatment[19]

Composition: Four patients with severe aphasia and limited verbal skills. Overall PICA scores for these patients ranged from the nineteenth to the thirty-third percentile.

Time postonset: All patients were at least 15 months postonset.

Amount of treatment: Patients were seen once per week for 90 minutes. Treatment effects were assessed over a 6-month period.

Objectives: Increase social interaction, increase recreational options, and promote generalization of communication skills across multiple settings.

Representative activities: Group members select recreational activity (e.g., bowling). Establish hierarchy of tasks leading to independent performance of the activity (e.g., keep score, seek out senior citizen rates, get shoes). Rehearse communication strategies used in the activity. Do the activity (outside the group) with group members performing all communication and only enlisting help from other group members. Debrief (e.g., identify successes, problems, and suggest ways of coping with future problems). The actual activity takes place outside the treatment room. Planning an activity, rehearsing communication strategies, assigning roles, and debriefing may extend over several in-house treatment sessions.

Results: Pre- and post-treatment comparisons showed the following: (1) Three of four patients made no change on their overall PICA score; (2) all patients showed pre- to post-treatment improvements on a functional measure, the Communicative Effectiveness Index (CETI)[20]; and (3) counts of discourse behaviors revealed greater variety of communicative acts, use of more questions, requests for assistance, and increased repairs.

Special features: This group is cofacilitated by a speech-language pathologist and a recreation therapist. Use of loose training techniques in planning, rehearsing, implementing, and debriefing. Sessions are task-oriented but unstructured, allowing the clinician to vary input to the patient and facilitating feedback to the patient from different sources.

Group Treatment for Globally Aphasic Individuals[21]

Composition: Patients with global aphasia.

Time postonset: No information provided.

Amount of treatment: The group met once per week for 1 hour.

Objectives: To (1) increase the appropriate use of residual expressive communication skills (e.g., vocal, verbal, gestural, nonverbal) during functional language activities; (2) increase auditory comprehension of salient, concrete, basic yes/no and informational questions, and verbal commands; and (3) encourage use of appropriate social/pragmatic behaviors during group.

Representative activities: Group members and clinicians look at and pass around large photographs of classic film stars (e.g., Clark Gable). Film stars are identified and their roles and films discussed. Clinicians ask group members basic yes/no and informational questions about the film stars and prompt members to pass the pictures around and vote about the film stars' attributes (e.g., talent, popularity, appeal). Clinicians promote the following skills: (1) turn-taking, (2) auditory comprehension of basic yes/no questions, (3) use of a variety of communicative acts, (4) social interaction, and (5) participation in voting.

Special features: Authors use a weekly checklist to assess group members' performance in the sessions. Completing the checklist involves assigning ratings (1 = never; 2 = poor; 3 = fair; 4 = good; 5 = normal) to the patient's behavior during the session (e.g., Did the patient attend to the activity?) and language-related behaviors (e.g., Did the patient follow the main ideas expressed by others?).

Intensive Group Treatment[22]

Composition: Five poststroke men, three with Broca's aphasia and two with mixed aphasia with respective ratings of 2, 1, 1, 2, and 3 on the Boston Diagnostic Aphasia Examination (BDAE) Severity Rating Scale.[23]

Time postonset: Patients were 24, 60, 14, 9, and 48 months postonset, respectively.

Amount of treatment: Patients were followed for 12 weeks: 4 weeks of no treatment, 4 weeks of intensive treatment, and 4 weeks of no treatment. In the intensive treatment period, subjects were seen for 10–15 hours per week, 5 days per week. The author reports that patients received a total of 85 hours of therapy during the intensive treatment period. Approximately 75% of this time was spent in group treatment; the remainder was spent in individual treatment.

Objectives: Objectives were to improve speech, a goal for all patients, as well as to improve expression through use of gestures, drawing, and writing. Patients were encouraged to communicate in any way possible within the group.

Representative activities: Group treatment sessions were described as "ongoing and flexible." Discussion topics were developed on a day-to-day basis as group interests emerged. Individual treatment activities involved picture naming facilitated by use of auditory semantic discrimination, word-to-picture matching, yes/no questioning, and verbal expression tasks prompted by *wh-* questions.

Results: Progress during the intensive treatment period was assessed with a variety of measures: short version of the CADL, the Bedside Evaluation Screening Test,[24] a picture-naming test, and a verbal expression measure. Every patient showed improvement on at least one test. The author concluded that a reasonable amount of improvement was achieved in a 1-month period of intensive treatment.

Group Treatment of Clients with Broca's Aphasia[25]

Composition: Ten patients (five men and five women) with Broca's aphasia. Patients ranged in age from 25 to 51 years (mean, 36 years). Severity of aphasia was measured with BDAE ratings.

Time postonset: Time postonset ranged from 18 to 130 months (mean, 51 months).

Amount of treatment: Treatment was described as intensive. Two groups of five subjects received 5 hours of speech therapy 5 days per week for 12 consecutive weeks. Twelve-week periods of nonintensive treatment preceded and followed the intensive treatment period. Nonintensive treatment was defined as individual treatment 1–2 hours per week, in some cases supplemented by a group therapy session.

Objectives: To compare the effects of intensive and nonintensive levels of conventional speech therapy intervention on the speech of well-motivated patients with chronic Broca's aphasia.

Representative activities: Treatment was delivered by a team of speech therapists. During the intensive program, patients lived in the hospital during the week in which they received 25 hours of therapy and went home on weekends. Treatment involved five programs: syntax, effective communication, word retrieval, articulation, and verbal memory. Selection and conduct of programs was individually determined on the basis of clinical assessment data. The purposes of each program were the following:

1. Syntax: To develop and stabilize verb forms with other clause, phrase, and word structures according to individual needs.

2. Effective communication: To use role-play to increase (a) efficiency of verbal interactions in different conversations, (b) initiation of speech, and (c) use of everyday phrases, and (d) awareness/anticipation of conversational sequences in social situations. Major themes were greetings, introductions, communication within and outside the home setting, and interview situations.

3. Word retrieval: To identify systematically and facilitate retrieval in lexical fields with which the individual had problems but showed potential for accurate word retrieval.

4. Articulation: Use of graded speech production tasks focusing on consonant singles, clusters, and vowels, as well as work on articulation rate, prosody, and sequencing.

5. Verbal memory program: To improve attention and increase short-term memory.

Results: All patients were assessed at the beginning of the first nonintensive period, at the beginning of the intensive period, at the end of the intensive period, and at the end of the second nonintensive period with the Functional Communication Profile[26] and the LARSP.[27] The only period in which the patients made any significant improvement was during the intensive treatment period. Improvements were significant for both measures. The authors conclude that intensive treatment courses are helpful to chronic, motivated patients with Broca's aphasia.

PSYCHOSOCIAL-FOCUSED GROUP TREATMENT FOR APHASIA

Aphasia and its resulting limitations on self-expression have serious and multiple psychosocial consequences. These psychosocial changes and stresses that occur for the aphasic person and his or her relatives affect all aspects of one's life: relationships, work, finances, leisure, mental health, and others.[28] Those concerned with minimizing or reducing the psychosocial consequences of aphasia recognize that aphasia is a chronic problem and that the members of the aphasic person's immediate environment (e.g., family, caregivers, and friends) may need as much support, education, and guidance as the patient does.[29–31] Psychosocially focused group treatment programs for aphasia endeavor to assist patients in forgetting about the aphasia and doing what is necessary to participate in life to the fullest extent in accordance with their preserved residuals.[32]

Preventing Social Dependence[33]

Composition: Thirty-four stroke patients, 19 men and 15 women (mean age, 48.7 years), who participated in a group rehabilitation program (Afa-Club) sponsored by the Cracow Speech Rehabilitation Club.

Time postonset: Not provided.

Amount of treatment: Weekly meetings for 30 months.

Objective: To restore social contacts, improve linguistic communication, and prevent social dependence.

Representative activities: This holistic approach to aphasia treatment involves a rehabilitation team (physician, neuropsychologist, speech-pathologist, social worker, and occupational therapist). Besides working to improve communication in the group, patients are encouraged to test their linguistic abilities in increasingly difficult situations: (1) simple, emotional situations at home; (2) more difficult situations at the Afa-Club; and (3) in the most difficult situations in their environment.

Results: The author concluded from examination of the data from several measures that the rehabilitation program was effective in improving communication, reducing anxiety, depression, and unfavorable reactions to disability. She indicated the program helped shape everyday activity, made patients active and self-dependent, and helped them take part in social activities.

Psychosocial-Oriented Group Approach with Chronic Aphasic Individuals[30]

Composition: An older group of four men and three women, 60–80 years old, and a younger group of five women and three men, 26–51 years of age. No information on severity of the patients' aphasia was provided.

Time postonset: Two to 5 years for the older group; 2–11 years for the younger group.

Amount of treatment: The older group met once per week for 2 hours with a psychologist and a speech therapist. The younger group met 22 times with a speech therapist.

Objectives: To learn to cope with aphasia and its inherent impairments, disabilities, and handicaps.

Representative activities: Treatment of the elderly group stressed "free interaction" and exchange about psychosocial burden and its impact as the main topic. Elements from communication oriented treatments (e.g., Promoting Aphasic Communicative Effectiveness) and memory training were also included in treatment, but these activities "gave way" as free interaction gained weight and importance and patients could talk about mutual experiences (e.g., holiday events) and problems (e.g., hemiparesis). The topics of illness and inherent fears of being left alone or dying were brought up by more than half of the elderly group.

Results: No objective results are provided. Observations by the authors suggest that the protected atmosphere of the groups allowed patients to develop and test new behavioral strategies and that groups contributed to increased competence and performance as well as to development of a higher, more realistic degree of self-esteem.

Special comments: The use of "free interaction" and discussion of coping strategies to reduce psychosocial burden was problematic because of the severe communicative deficits of some younger group members. In the younger group, the therapist took a more directive role. Members preferred to work on communication, interactions, and to minimize psychological impairments (e.g., attention deficits) to avoid difficult or controversial topics. Issues of psychosocial burden were not discussed until the final treatment sessions. The authors use this finding as support for having separate groups for younger and older patients.

Innovative Therapy Program for Aphasic Patients and Their Relatives[34]

Composition: Eleven patients with aphasia ranging in age from 39 to 62 years (mean, 50 years) and seven family members were randomly selected from a list of applicants. Patients with global aphasia were not involved in this study.

Time postonset: Not provided.

Amount of therapy: Participants attended a 5-day intensive course held at a boarding school in a small town.

Objectives: To examine the psychological, linguistic, and neurologic effects of an intensive 5-day informational and psychotherapeutic program provided to aphasic patients and their families.

Representative activities: Participants met in four groups led by a speech teacher. Members of the same family were placed in separate groups. Groups discussed news from the daily paper, objects that patients brought to the session, music, and poems, and they sang. In smaller groups, aphasic patients worked on reading, writing, and naming drills. Participants also listened to lectures, went on various excursions, and spent time in evening discussion groups comparing their everyday problems and coming up with new ideas for solving their personal difficulties.

One at a time the family broke out of group meetings to meet with the psychologist for examination and family therapy. Within these interview sessions, spouses reported observations on specific abilities of the aphasic partner (e.g., memory and emotional self-regulation) and completed a test battery. Family therapy focused on relationships in the family, and the psychologist explored changes in relationships that occurred because of the aphasia. Patients were also examined neurologically and administered an aphasia test and selected items from the BDAE.

Results: Course participants met 1 year after the course for re-evaluation. Those participating in re-evaluation (nine aphasics and six family members) were found to make positive changes psychologically and interpersonally, but not linguistically and neurologically.

Family Therapy in Families with an Aphasic Member[35]

Composition: Participants were members of the Swedish Aphasia Association. Degree and type of aphasia for the patient participants varied. Patients with a diagnosis of global aphasia, those experiencing melancholy, those with a noninvolved family, and those directly involved in other training/psychotherapy programs were not included in the project. A total of 37 family members and 22 aphasic patients were involved in the study. Five aphasic patients and nine family members dropped out before the program started.

Time postonset: Not stated.

Amount of therapy: In all cases, therapy was limited to a minimum of two and a maximum of six sessions over a short period.

Objectives: Aims of family therapy can be summarized as follows: (1) to explore the cognitive and emotional aspects of the family before, during, and after a family member becomes aphasic; (2) to teach the family about the handicap of aphasia and typical reactions to it; (3) to encourage emotional sharing in the family (e.g., acting out grief, anger); (4) to confront common issues and introduce open communication about delicate issues (e.g., sex); (5) to encourage aphasic persons to explain what kind of help they want from family members (e.g., filling in words); (6) to teach family members how to time interactions differently; (7) to teach family members how to notice nonverbal communication efforts and to check and clarify interpretations; (8) to teach family members to use special feedback techniques to compensate for motor speech disorders; and (9) to discourage family members from providing formal linguistic training to the patient.

Representative activities: The information is too extensive to be included in this synopsis. For representative activities associated with the program, the reader should consult the reference list.[35, 36]

Results: All participants completed a questionnaire 6 months before and 6 months after receiving family therapy. Responses to questions targeting emotional, behavioral, social, communicative, and medical changes occurring as a consequence of family therapy were scored on a five-point scale. Results revealed that depression, emotional isolation, impatience, and social isolation were diminished in the aphasic patients after family therapy; both aphasic patients and the family members increased their knowledge about the handicap of aphasia. A 10-year follow-up of eight young patients who participated in the program found that patients reported greater satisfaction with life after having participated in the educational program.[37]

Social Support Group for Spouses of Aphasic Partners[38]

Composition: Ten aphasic patients ranging in age from 53 to 66 years (mean, 60 years) and their spouses participated in the study. Most of the aphasic patients had global, conduction, or Broca's aphasia.

Time postonset: This period ranged from 2 to 23 months (mean, 9 months).

Amount of treatment: Only the spouses were involved in the social support group. This group met weekly in the evenings for a 2-hour period for 12 weeks.

Objective: To satisfy the psychological needs of spouses of aphasic people by providing information, enhancing psychological adjustment, and initiating strategies to improve functional communication.

Representative activities: Sessions involved structured educational programs (e.g., videotapes on aphasia, role of the physiotherapist, social worker talking on support agencies, holiday advice for the aphasic person) and open-discussion sessions during which specific issues could be addressed in the group. All sessions allowed participants to discuss issues with the speech therapist, the invited speaker, and other members of the group.

Results: Two measures of psychological well-being were used to assess the effectiveness of the program, the Goldberg General Health Questionnaire[39] and the Mulhall Personality Questionnaire Rapid Scaling Technique.[40] Only five of the spouses attended the sessions regularly. Regular attendees showed significant improvement on tests of social dysfunction, somatic symptoms, and anxiety as well as on a broad measure of psychological well-being. Their aphasic partners also evidenced some functional improvement in communication.

Opening Doors: An Alternative Family Education Program[41-42]

Composition: This group consisted of 139 individuals (patients with aphasia and family members) who attended a follow-up, intensive aphasia program at a residential aphasia center. Data on severity and type of aphasia are not available.

Time postonset: All patients with aphasia are described as being chronic.

Amount of therapy: The authors describe this intervention as a 2-day family education conference aimed at assessing the long-term psychosocial effects of persons with aphasia and their family members. Three years of program data are reported by the authors.

Objectives: Program goals address needs of patients with aphasia and their families. These goals are to (1) provide opportunities to gain a better understanding of the physical, emotional, and psychosocial consequences of aphasia; (2) review resources for communication, transportation, vocational and avocational pursuits, and assistive devices; and (3) create a forum for participants to share their experiences and learn from one another.

Representative activities: The most common topical areas covered in this educational program include communication issues, intimacy and sexuality, participant discussion groups, parenting, vocational issues, coping, driving, and volunteering.

Results: The Community Integration Questionnaire (CIQ), an instrument designed to assess social integration skills, was used to measure the success of the Opening Doors program. The CIQ has three subscales:

1. The home integration subscale assesses which member of the home is responsible for basic activities (e.g., child care, banking).
2. The social integration subscale evaluates the frequency and independence with which the individual encounters persons outside the home.
3. The productivity subscale assesses the individual's vocational status.

Scores on the CIQ range from 0 to 29 points. More points suggest greater independence. CIQ results are available for 50 aphasic adults who completed at least one of the Opening Doors programs, 10 other adults with aphasia and family members who completed two program sessions, and a control group of 12 adults with aphasia and their caregivers who inquired about Opening Doors but did not participate. Pre- and post-CIQ results were not significantly different. Participation in Opening Doors, however, did make a significant difference on the social integration scale for subjects enrolled in the program, but not for the control subjects.

A Unique Method for Follow-Up of Aphasic Patients[43]

Composition: Patients discharged from aphasia therapy. The authors report that patients attending the sessions cluster into three groups on the severity rating scale of the BDAE: (1) males with BDAE severity ratings between 3 and 5; (2) females with ratings between 3 and 5; and (3) men and women with BDAE scores from 0 to 2 and severe limitations.

Time postonset: No specific information is provided.

Amount of therapy: Group sessions are considered "alumni reunions." The reunions are held on a Saturday afternoon to follow-up on aphasic patients who have been dismissed from treatment.

Objectives: Speech-language pathologists use these social gatherings to determine how former patients are adjusting to the residuals of aphasia and to assess the use of communication skills in an informal setting.

Representative activities: The reunions have three segments: (1) a reception with refreshments where speech-language pathologists interact with the patients and perform their informal assessments; (2) a "shared experience" with family members meeting in a larger group to review the purpose of the reunion and to hear an informational presentation from a guest speaker; and (3) a segment with a "psychosocial focus" when caregivers are allowed to speak more openly of the difficulties in living with a person with aphasia.

Results: No data are provided.

Group Therapy for Severely Aphasic and Hemiplegic Patients[44]

Composition: Six patients with severe expressive aphasia. Four of the patient's spouses participated in the group program.

Time postonset: Aphasic group members ranged from 6 months to 3 years.

Amount of therapy: The group met 1 hour per week for 1 year without interruption. Group sessions were attended by two speech therapists, a psychiatrist, a physiatrist, patients, and spouses.

Objective: To examine the use of group therapy as a therapeutic tool to explore, reinforce, and maintain the positive motivation necessary to maximize rehabilitation.

Representative activities: Over a year of treatment this psychotherapeutically focused group evolved through three stages: (1) an initial period of anxiety, confusion, and difficulty communicating with each other; (2) a period marked by complaints, misgivings, and disappointments about the home situation, the hospital environment, and social circumstances; and (3) a period of mutual understanding, friendliness, and better adaptation to the home, the hospital, and outside settings.

Results: The group was thought to be helpful in the following ways: (1) developing a more realistic outlook on illnesses; (2) allowing venting of hostile feelings stemming from increased dependency; (3) allowing members to see "others like me;" (4) allowing the speech therapist to intersperse short speech lessons throughout the group sessions; (5) providing a setting in which conflicts could be acted out in a controlled fashion; and (6) reducing social isolation.

Community-Based Aphasia Program[45]

Composition: The York-Durham Aphasia Centre (YDAC) is a community-based program for persons with aphasia and their families. Aphasic patients at all levels of severity participate in the program. Five or six groups containing five aphasic patients operate simultaneously. A caregiver support group, led by a social worker, meets at the same time as the communication groups.

Time postonset: All patients are chronic.

Amount of therapy: The communication group program is offered twice per week for a half day. This program is delivered by trained volunteers with support and guidance from speech-language pathologists and a communication disorders assistant.

Objectives: The program addresses the long-term communicative and social needs of persons with severe and chronic aphasia and their families. The objectives of the program are numerous and diverse. The philosophy of the YDAC is that persons with aphasia have a fundamental right to be able to express their needs, feelings, and thoughts so as to reveal competencies hidden by aphasia.[46] Additional information on the YDAC program can also be found in publications by its founder and director[47, 48] and in an informational handbook published by YDAC (now called the *Pat Arato Aphasia Center*).[49]

Representative activities: Volunteers facilitate opportunities for aphasic patients to exchange ideas, learn adaptive skills to improve communication effectiveness, and make friends. The program stresses adaptive techniques to assist group members in conversing: drawing, gesturing, role-playing, writing, and using keywords. The caregiver program provides family members an environment needed for reflection, sharing experiences, and problem solving, as well as assists them in learning to cope with their new roles and regain a sense of well-being in their lives.

Results: Improvement in psychological well-being of 35 patients and 12 family members participating in the YDAC program was assessed over a 6-month period using a modification of Ryff's Psychological Well-Being Index.[50] Both patients and family members were found to improve on five of six dimensions of psychological well-being.

Special features: Positive comments on the YDAC program have come from several sources.[29, 51–55] Many see this community resource as a model for long-term treatment of aphasia and its psychosocial sequelae. Research on the efficacy and effectiveness of the YDAC program is currently under way.

Communicative Autonomy Treatment[56]

Composition: Four patients (two men and two women) ranging in age from 47 to 76 years with severe aphasia. Severity of aphasia was determined by WAB AQs. The four participants had the following scores: 9.2, 24.4, 42.1, and 30.7.

Time postonset: Patients ranged from 8 to 99 months postonset.

Amount of treatment: Treatment was conducted at a university clinic. Treatment involved thirty 90-minute sessions over a 9-month period. The patient's spouses also participated in the treatment sessions as did student therapists assigned to each patient.

Objectives: To teach patients to use augmentative communication tools and strategies to achieve personalized conversational goals.

Representative activities: Group members and conversational partners completed a Q-sort task to choose least and most preferred communication topics. Participants customized the general sort categories based on personal needs (e.g., sharing small talk about day-to-day activities with friends from church) and developed personal goal attainment scales for each personalized topic. During the treatment sessions, participants, students, and family members met for 45 minutes in a large group, where they engaged in semistructured discussion. This session was followed by individual or small group sessions, where individual or pairs of participants worked on personal goals. Individual and partner training sessions were scheduled for some participants apart from the group sessions.

Results: All participants demonstrated the ability to achieve self-selected communication goals, to improve overall functional communication as measured by the CETI, and to resume prestroke activity level as assessed by an activity level scale.

Building a Community Aphasia Group[57]

Composition: Patients with mild-to-severe aphasia (WAB AQ scores 35–92) who live at home, in residential settings, or in skilled nursing facilities. Volunteers (graduate students in speech-language pathology, undergraduate students in social work, biology, and communication disorders, community volunteers) and speech-language pathologists are responsible for the program. Support for the program comes from the health care system's rehabilitation team, which includes several professionals.

Time postonset: Patients ranged from 6 days to 12 years postonset. Most participants, however, were patients with chronic aphasia (80%) who were finished with individual treatment.

Amount of treatment: Currently, this health care system has four ongoing groups. Three groups are for patients with mild, moderate, and severe aphasia; one group is for caregivers. This program began within the Luther Midelfort Mayo Health System in March of 1997 as a means of meeting long-term needs of persons with aphasia. It appears that patients are free to attend groups as they see fit. An average of seven patients attended each group during the first year.

Objectives: This unique program has developed short- and long-range goals. The first year of the program focused on staff training, recruitment and training of volunteers, and the development of a database for patients and caregivers. In the second year of the program, the investigators will optimize the delivery system through research activities.

Representative activities: Authentic conversation in natural contexts with communication partners who provide "ramps" to ensure that information is exchanged and understood. Treatment is conversation-based. Patients are encouraged to use strategies that facilitate information exchange. Outcomes are measured with linguistic and psychosocial measures.

Special features: This new program represents an important step in aphasia treatment. Specifically, this is the formation of a collaborative partnership between a health care system, the Luther-Midelfort System, education, and the community to provide necessary resources and services for persons with aphasia to maintain social connections. This type of partnership represents a major departure from the use of medical model resources that are limited. Collaborative partnerships offer a means of involving people with aphasia in the community outside of the health care system.

City Dysphasic Group[58]

Composition: Since its inception in 1994, 100 persons with aphasia (58 men, 42 women) have been referred to the group program. Severity of aphasia was described as mild, moderate, and severe for 24, 47, and 29 patients, respectively. Participants resided in the greater London area.

Time postonset: Twenty-two patients started the program before 6 months postonset; 29 began the program between 7 and 12 months postonset; 13 began the program after 3 years postonset.

Amount of treatment: Typically, patients attend the center 2 full days per week. In those 2 days, they receive six or seven group sessions and one or two individual treatment periods.

Objectives: Activities at the City Dysphasic Group address three major components of aphasia: (1) language and communication, (2) confidence and self-identity, and (3) coping with lifestyle changes.

Representative activities: Language and communication goals appear to be addressed in a traditional fashion with work on improving speech and finding words, improving reading and writing skills, supplementing speech with gesture and drawing, and encouraging the use of alternative means of communication. Confidence and self-identity are improved by promoting advocacy and assertiveness in the patient with aphasia, counseling, and improving self-esteem. The center provides a counseling service (eight sessions per week) and participants attend an average of six counseling sessions yearly. Lifestyle changes and coping with the changes brought about by aphasia are addressed by training conversation partners; providing support for caregivers; improving patients' access to education, work, and leisure activities; and educating society in general about disability.

Special features: This novel program has a long track record of success, and its training and research activities are noteworthy. An important "back up" feature of this program is its supplementary group programs. These include a counseling service, a conversation group for patients who have been dismissed from formal treatment, a self-help group, a self-advocacy group, and a caregiver's group. Unique also is that the developers of the City Dysphasic Group have actively and successfully sought funding for the program.

TRANSITIONAL GROUPS

Transitional groups provide support and guidance for the stroke patient as he or she moves through the various stages of the rehabilitation process: acute care to rehabilitation program and rehabilitation program to home. Group membership includes not only patients with aphasia, but those with other cognitive-communicative (e.g., right hemisphere communication disorder, dysarthria), physical (e.g., hemiplegia), and behavioral (e.g., abulia, emotional liability) manifestations of stroke and its many syndromes. Although transitional groups may contain patients with communicative problems such as aphasia, their purpose is not to work on communication per se, but rather to facilitate discharge planning for the patient and movement from one setting to another.

Transitional groups can therefore be expected to change in composition from week to week as new patients are admitted to or exit the program. In most health care organizations, transitional groups have a short-term duration. These groups serve multiple purposes: imparting information, counseling, and problem solving. Mostly, these purposes reflect the philosophy of the sponsoring program. Leadership positions in these groups are often assumed by social workers and other mental health professionals with interest in strokes.

Discharge Planning and Community Involvement[59]

Composition: Right and left hemisphere stroke patients in a rehabilitation program are referred to the discharge-planning group (DPG) as they approach maximum hospital benefit, usually after they have gone home for a trial weekend. After the patient goes home, he or she is placed in the community involvement group (CIG).

Time postonset: No information provided.

Amount of therapy: The two active group treatment programs, DPG and CIG, last 4–6 months. Patients attend these groups when they are receiving outpatient therapies. After discharge from active therapies, the patients attend a monthly stroke club meeting.

Objectives: The DPG is issue-oriented. The goal is to get the patient to think of what life will be like when he or she goes home. The aim of the CIG is to help the patient accept a lifestyle altered by stroke and to develop appropriate alternatives.

Representative activities: "When you were home for the weekend, how did you get from the living room to the bathroom?" or "What did you do when the telephone rang?" are the types of questions that patients are asked when meeting in the DPG. Within the CIG, the patient might focus on changing his or her role within the family structure. For example, a male patient whose wife needed to work outside the home might be encouraged to assume household duties he considered to be "women's work."

Results: No objective results are provided. The author does, however, report that right hemisphere damaged patients without aphasia have more problems in the DPG and CIG groups and in adjusting to community placements than left hemisphere damaged aphasic patients. Primary reasons for this difference appear to be neglect and inappropriate behaviors.

Short-Term Group Treatment[60]

Composition: Three groups of patients with mixed etiologies (e.g., right hemisphere CVA, left hemisphere tumor). The average age of the group members was 50 years. Nineteen of 21 group members had some form of mobility. Group members had to have sufficient language and comprehension to participate in the group; however, no information of severity of these deficits is provided.

Time postonset: Determining when patients started the group is not possible, but the impression is that they joined shortly after having had a stroke.

Amount of therapy: An average of seven patients attended the group meetings. All patients had to commit to attending at least three meetings. The number of meetings for each group was six.

Objectives: These groups were discussion groups led jointly by a social worker and a psychiatric registrar. Therapists documented the themes and problems discussed within the groups, which focused on physical (e.g., mobility, driving, housework) and psychological (e.g., expectations about progress, communication, reasons for strokes) issues related to stroke.

Representative activities: Apparently, operations of the group were determined by what "came up" within the meeting. For example, a female patient expressed her feelings about the inadequacy of her husband and children in coping with household chores. She described her anger and frustration at not being able to do her chores and at having to refrain from criticizing. Other patients with similar concerns then joined in this discussion.

Results: Follow-up questionnaires were sent to participants 3 months after the end of treatment. Patients returned 13 of 23 questionnaires: 10 patients indicated that the groups had been useful and helpful on a three-point evaluation scale. The primary reason for positive comments was that the group had allowed patients to share problems, reducing isolation and increasing self-confidence. Therapists' evaluation of the short-term group treatment program indicated that it helped them learn about problems patients faced and discover themes that ran consistently through all groups.

Psychotherapy with Stroke Patients in the Immediate Recovery Phase[61]

Composition: Twenty-two stroke patients who had been transferred from an intensive care unit of a stroke unit to the subacute ward. A minimum of four patients were needed in a group, and patients had to be capable of some degree of verbal communication.

Time postonset: Groups began relatively soon after stroke.

Amount of treatment: Patients were seen in two open-ended groups. Groups met 5 days per week for 30-minute sessions. Ten patients (three women and seven men) attended 15 sessions. Twelve patients (11 men and 1 woman) attended 11 meetings.

Objectives: (1) Help patients identify the nature of the crisis brought about by the stroke. (2) Assist patients in expression of feelings about the crisis. (3) Encourage patients to explore new coping strategies. (4) Assist patients in re-entering the social world.

Representative activities: Discussion of patient-focused anxieties about future unknowns such as having another stroke, regaining use of a paretic limb, and planning for discharge occupied early meetings. In midphase meetings, after patients had come to know one another, more sensitive issues were discussed (e.g., sexual functioning, loss of control, social and physical losses) and patients were able to voice feelings of anger and frustration before becoming more realistic about discharge and problems to follow. During the final meetings, group members had been granted weekend visits. Feelings of confusion, ambivalence, apprehension, and how patients thought they would be accepted by "well" people were discussed.

Results: Program effectiveness was evaluated by means of a questionnaire sent to 21 patients who participated in the group program. Only eight questionnaires were returned. Responses indicated that the group discussion helped patients understand their illness and its effects and to accept its inherent limitations. Responses also indicated that group meetings helped them feel more comfortable in the hospital, less alone, and they occupied time. Five of eight patients said the group helped them to cope with depression.

Special features: The authors point out that daily ward discussion groups allowed patients with strokes to become acquainted with each other, and fostered subsequent socialization on the ward. Patients developed a sense of community among themselves, their families, and the staff.

REFERENCES

1. Kearns K. Group Therapy for Aphasia: Theoretical and Practical Considerations. In R Chapey (ed), Language Intervention Strategies in Adult Aphasia (3rd ed). Baltimore: Williams & Wilkins, 1994;304.
2. Kearns K, Simmons NN. Group Therapy for Aphasia: A Survey of Veterans Administration Medical Centers. In RH Brookshire (ed), Clinical Aphasiology Conference Proceedings. Minneapolis: BRK, 1985;176.
3. Wertz RT, Collins MH, Weiss D, et al. Veterans Administration cooperative study on aphasia. A comparison of individual and group treatment. J Speech Hear Res 1981;24:580.

4. Porch BE. The Porch Index of Communicative Ability. Palo Alto, CA: Consulting Psychologists, 1967.

5. Vogel D. Group Treatment for Aphasia: A Panel Discussion. In R Brookshire (ed), Clinical Aphasiology Conference Proceedings. Minneapolis: BRK, 1981;144.

6. Avent JR. Group treatment in aphasia using a cooperative learning method. J Med Speech-Lang Pathol 1997;5:9.

7. Kertesz A. Western Aphasia Battery. New York: Grune & Stratton, 1982.

8. Avent JR. Introduction to Cooperative Group Treatment. In J Avent (ed), Manual of Cooperative Group Treatment for Aphasia. Boston: Butterworth–Heinemann, 1997;1.

9. Bollinger RL, Musson ND, Holland AL. A study of group communication intervention with chronically aphasic persons. Aphasiology 1993;7:301.

10. Holland AL. Communicative Abilities in Daily Living. Baltimore: University Park Press, 1980.

11. Radonjic V, Rakkuscek N. Group therapy to encourage communication ability in aphasia patients. Aphasiology 1991;5:451.

12. Elman RJ, Burnstein-Ellis E. Effectiveness of Group Communication Treatment for Individuals with Chronic Aphasia: Results on Communicative and Linguistic Measures. Paper presented at the Clinical Aphasiology Conference, Newport, RI, June 1996.

13. DiSimoni F, Kieth R, Darley F. Prediction of PICA overall score by short version of the test. J Speech Hear Res 1980;23:511.

14. Aten J, Caliguri M, Holland A. The efficacy of functional communication therapy for chronic aphasic patients. J Speech Hear Disord 1872;47:93.

15. Marshall RC. Problem-focused group treatment for clients with mild aphasia. Am J Speech-Lang Pathol 1993;3:31.

16. Klingman S. Cooperative Group Treatment for Mild Aphasia. In J Avent (ed), Manual of Cooperative Group Treatment for Aphasia. Boston: Butterworth–Heinemann, 1997;19.

17. Kaplan E, Goodglass H, Weintraub S. The Boston Naming Test. Philadelphia: Lea & Febiger, 1983.

18. Fratalli C, Thompson C, Holland A, et al. Functional Assessment of Communication Skills for Adults. Rockville, MD: American Speech-Language-Hearing Association, 1995.

19. Fox L. Recreation Focused Treatment for Generalization of Language Skills in Aphasic Patients. Paper presented at the American Speech-Language-Hearing Association Convention, Seattle, November 1990.

20. Lomas J, Pickard L, Bester S, et al. The communicative effectiveness index: development and psychometric evaluation of a functional measure for adult aphasia. J Speech Hear Disord 1989;54:113.

21. Erskine B, Moody CS, Rau MT. Group Treatment for Globally Aphasic Individuals. Paper presented at the Oregon and Washington Speech and Hearing Association, Seattle, October 1987.

22. Makenzie C. Four weeks of intensive therapy followed by four weeks of no treatment. Aphasiology 1991;5:435

23. Goodglass H, Kaplan E. Boston Diagnostic Aphasia Examination. Philadelphia: Lea & Febiger, 1983.

24. West JF, Sands EA. Bedside Evaluation and Screening Test for Aphasia. New York: Prentice-Hall, 1989.

25. Brindley P, Copeland M, Demain C, Martyn P. A comparison of the speech of ten chronic Broca's aphasic patients following intensive and non-intensive periods of therapy. Aphasiology 1989;3:695.
26. Sarno M. The Functional Communication Profile Manual of Directions. Rehabilitation Monographs 42. New York: New York University, 1969;1.
27. Crystal D, Fletcher P, Garman M. The Grammatical Analysis of Language Disability. London: Edward Arnold, 1976;1.
28. Brumfitt S. Losing your sense of self: what aphasia can do. Aphasiology 1993;7:569.
29. Lyon J. Coping with Aphasia. San Diego: Singular, 1998.
30. Johannsen-Horbach H, Wenz C, Funfgeld M, et al. Psychosocial Aspects in the Treatment of Adult Aphasics and their Families: A Group Approach in Germany. In A Holland, M Forbes (eds), Aphasia Treatment: World Perspectives. London: Chapman, 1993;319.
31. LeDorze GE, Brassard C. A description of consequences of aphasia on aphasic persons and their relatives and friends based on the WHO model of chronic diseases. Aphasiology 1995;9:295.
32. Lyon J. Communication use and participation in life for adults with aphasia in natural settings: the scope of the problem. Am J Speech-Lang Pathol 1993;3:7.
33. Pachalska MK. Prevention of the state of social dependence of patients afflicted with aphasia. Am J Soc Psychiatry 1982;2:51.
34. Bornstein P, Linell S, Wahrborg P. An innovative therapeutic program for aphasia patients and their relatives. Scand J Rehabil Med 1987;19:51.
35. Wahrborg P, Bornstein P. Family therapy in families with an aphasic member. Aphasiology 1989;3:93.
36. Hall AD, Fagen RE. Definition of System. In LV Bertalannfy and A Rappaport (eds), General Systems Yearbook 1. New York: Society for General Systems Research, 1956.
37. Wahrborg P, Borenstein P, Linell E, et al. Ten-year follow-up of young aphasic participants in a 34-week course at a folk high school. Aphasiology 1997;11:709.
38. Rice B, Paull A, Miller DJ. An evaluation of a social support group for spouses of aphasic partners. Aphasiology 1987;1:247.
39. Goldberg D. Manual of General Health Questionnaire. Windsor, UK: NFER-Nelson, 1978.
40. Mulhall DJ. Manual for Personal Questionnaire Rapid Scaling Technique. Windsor: NFER-Nelson, 1978.
41. Hinckley JJ, Packard M, Bardach LG. Alternative family education programming for adults with chronic aphasia. Top Stroke Rehabil 1995;2:53.
42. Hinckley JJ, Packard M, Cowels S, et al. Impacting the Psychosocial Effects of Aphasia through Family Education Programs. Paper presented at the American Speech-Language-Hearing Association Convention, Boston, November 1997.
43. Mogil S, Bloom D, Gray L, Lefkowitz N. A Unique Method for the Follow-up of Aphasic Patients. In R Brookshire (ed), Clinical Aphasiology Conference Proceedings. Minneapolis: BRK, 1978;314.
44. Redinger RA, et al. Group therapy in the rehabilitation of the severely aphasic and hemiplegic in the late stages. Scand J Rehabil Med 1971;3:89.
45. Hoen B, Thelander M, Worsley J. Improvement in psychological well-being of people with aphasia and their families: evaluation of a community-based program. Aphasiology 1997;11:681.

46. Kagan A. Supported conversation for adults with aphasia: methods and resources for training conversation partners. Aphasiology 1998;12:816.
47. Kagan A. Revealing the competencies of aphasic adults through conversation: a challenge to health professionals. Top Stroke Rehabil 1995;2:1
48. Kagan A, Gailey G. Functional Is Not Enough: Training Conversation Partners for Aphasic Adults. In A Holland, M Forbes (eds), Aphasia Treatment: World Perspectives. London: Chapman, 1993;199.
49. York-Durham Aphasia Centre. Aphasia—A New Life. Toronto: Coopershill, 1994;1.
50. Ryff CD. Beyond Ponce de Leon and life satisfaction: new directions in quest of successful aging. Int J Behav Dev 1989;12:35.
51. Simmons-Mackie N. Supported conversation for adults with aphasia. Aphasiology 1998;12:831.
52. Holland A. Why can't clinicians talk to aphasic adults? Aphasiology 1998;12:844.
53. Penn C. Clinician-researcher dilemmas: comment on "supported conversation for adults with aphasia." Aphasiology 1998;12:839.
54. Byng S, Parr S. Breaking new ground in familiar territory: a response to "supported conversation for adults with aphasia" by Aura Kagan. Aphasiology 1998;12:847.
55. Marshall RC. An introduction to supported conversation for adults with aphasia: perspectives, problems, possibilities. Aphasiology 1998;12:811.
56. Fox L, Fried-Oken M. Trial Implementation of Communicative Autonomy Treatment in a Group Environment: A Case Study. Unpublished manuscript.
57. Pound C. Power, partnerships, and practicalities: developing cost-effective support services for living with aphasia. Paper presented at the Clinical Aphasiology Conference, Asheville, NC, June 1998.
58. Hintgen T, Clark MB, Radichel T. Development of a community-based aphasia program. Poster session at the Clinical Aphasiology Conference, Asheville, NC, June 1998.
59. West J. Group Treatment for Aphasia: A Panel Discussion. In R Brookshire (ed), Clinical Aphasiology Conference Proceedings. Minneapolis: BRK, 1981;149.
60. Bucher J, Smith E, Gillespie C. Short-term group therapy for stroke patients in a rehabilitation centre. Br J Med Psych 1984;57:283.
61. Oradei DM, Waite NS. Group psychotherapy with stroke patients during the immediate recovery phase. Am J Orthopsychiatry 1974;44:386.

8

Group Treatment Activities

Some years ago, after an American Speech-Language-Hearing Association (ASHA) convention presentation on management of aphasia, the audience was asked to submit questions to the session moderator. The moderator read the questions aloud for the audience to hear. Members of a panel composed of clinical aphasiologists answered the questions and discussed them with the audience. The one question I remember is the following: "Why don't you stop giving us all the theoretical stuff and just tell us what to do with our patients?"

No one can tell a clinician exactly what to do with an aphasic patient in a group or an individual situation. What clinicians do depends on an evaluation of many factors and interactive variables. Carrying out a specific treatment activity to maximize communication effectiveness is usually easier if the group is homogenous, but selecting the path to follow in treatment remains a complex endeavor. Those individual aphasic patients who make up any group are as different as snowflakes.[1]

The lengthy synopsis on group treatment programs provided in Chapter 7 gives some indication of the broad range of activities used in different group situations. In this chapter, I provide more specific information on group treatment activities that appear particularly well-suited to this therapeutic endeavor. Again, I wish to point out that what is presented here is not all-inclusive. Also, the activities reviewed here were not originally intended to be used in aphasia treatment groups, but in my opinion they can be used in this fashion. After each activity, I have interjected a comment or two as to how the activity might be used in a group situation.

STRUCTURED TELEVISION VIEWING

Structured television viewing group treatment (STVGT)[2] is a procedure designed to facilitate understanding and expression of communication

Table 8.1
Structured television viewing group treatment (STVGT) protocol.

---

1. The speech-language pathologist establishes a viewing strategy: who, what, where, and when?
2. The content is established with a 2- to 10-minute preliminary viewing.
3. The group provides key information, and the speech-language pathologist writes the information on the blackboard.
4. The group reviews the watched segment with attention to key elements.
5. The group relates the information.
6. The group predicts the events to follow based on previous viewing.
7. The 2- to 10-minute segment is viewed a third time.
8. The group recalls the main events of the segment.
9. Predictions are verified through the review of segments.
10. Additional segments are viewed with recall, prediction, and verification procedures used.
11. The entire episode is viewed.
12. Group discussion of plausibility of events, what they might change, and how they feel about the issues that were brought up.

Source: Reprinted with permission from RL Bollinger, ND Muson, AL Holland. A study of group communication intervention with chronically aphasic persons. Aphasiology 1993;7:301.

intents of television programs. Television programs for viewing are selected on the basis of continuity of characters and content (e.g., "Murphy Brown"). Programs have identifiable characters, contextually relevant dialogue, and predictable story lines. In STVGT, the clinician encourages patients to use a viewing strategy (e.g., watching for key elements including people, action, time, and places). The duration of the program segments viewed is tailored to fit patients' attention spans and typically ranges from 2 to 10 minutes. After viewing a program segment, the group and the therapist engage in a discussion focused on the identification of key elements of the program (e.g., communicative attributes, facial expression, body language, expletives, idioms). Table 8.1 provides a protocol for STVGT.

COMMENTARY

Given the amount of time Americans spend watching television (news, sports, situation comedies), can anything less be expected from persons with aphasia? STVGT shows how this national pastime can become a productive communicative activity for persons with aphasia. Once a strategy for STVGT has been taught, group members might be given homework assignments (e.g., watch a portion

Table 8.2
Phases of dollhouse project used in transdisciplinary group treatment.

Phase I: developing a plan
   Access resources (e.g., phone books, phone, funds, transportation) to locate
      stores that carry the dollhouse
Phase II: the purchase
   Use information obtained through community resources to comparison
      shop and make the best decision
Phase III: groundbreaking
   Identify foreman, whose first responsibility is to develop a plan and delegate
      tasks to include all patients
Phase IV: construction
   Modify construction process to promote teamwork and to incorporate
      various strengths and barriers of all patients
Phase V: finishing touches
   Finish construction project, including painting, interior decorating, and
      landscaping
Phase VI: ribbon cutting
   Donate project to children's organization of patients' choosing

---

of the news) and asked to prepare reports on what they learned for
the next group meeting.

DOLLHOUSE PROJECT

Jenkins and others illustrate how a group project, the building of a
dollhouse, can be used to help adults with acquired neurogenic disorders work on cognitive-communication skills in rehabilitation settings.[3] Three transdisciplinary cognitive skills groups (two to eight
patients) met two to three times weekly at different sites to work on
dollhouse projects. This construction project was divided into six
phases shown in Table 8.2. The authors suggest that participants work
together to research and plan, purchase the materials for, and build
the structure. Cognitive-communicative skills believed to benefit from
these activities include planning, problem solving, memory, auditory
comprehension, reading comprehension, verbal expression, and written expression.

COMMENTARY
   The dollhouse project, as described by its authors, is carried out over
   several group treatment sessions. Related, but shorter group projects,

may be accomplished in a single group session. Possible projects might include completing simple assembly tasks with written instructions (e.g., putting together a barbecue), learning how to operate a new piece of equipment (e.g., a new camera), repairing broken items, and performing similar day-to-day tasks. One of my groups spent an entire session figuring out how to extract a cork that had somehow become immersed in an expensive bottle of wine. They devised a unique vacuum system, removed the cork, and saved the wine.

REMINISCENCE

Reminiscence therapy taps a person's ability to recall and converse about topics, people, places, and events experienced in earlier times. Harris published an excellent paper on this subject that shows how reminiscence therapy can be used in group treatment of adults with aphasia, mild-moderate cognitive impairments, and elderly persons with intact communication skills.[4] Reminiscence therapy is based on "life review theory" and the fact that senior citizens can often make specific references to past life events, particularly those with autobiographic importance.[5] In her paper, Harris advocates using this approach in small groups (six to eight persons). She recommends that treatment focus on "event" (e.g., Roaring '20s), "calendar" (e.g., Fourth of July), "ladder of life" (e.g., teen years), or "historical timeline" (e.g., news on the day one was born) topics and avoid topics that are more controversial. Table 8.3 presents a sample of a reminiscence group activity.

COMMENTARY

Reminiscence is a popular group treatment approach in long-term care settings, but this methodology can be equally useful in group treatment of aphasia.[6] A long-standing axiom of aphasia treatment is that patients communicate better when topics of discussion are familiar and relate to past experiences. Reminiscence therapy fits well into this paradigm.

COOPERATIVE GROUP TREATMENT

The basics of cooperative group treatment (CGT) were described in Chapter 7.[7] In this treatment approach, two aphasic patients alternate roles of recaller and facilitator. The recaller retells a target story read earlier by the therapist. The facilitator cues, corrects, and adds omitted information as needed. Treatment stimuli are narrative and procedural stories similar to the example given in Figure 8.1. Stories are adjusted for length

Table 8.3
Example of a reminiscence group activity, with the theme, "It's Off to Work I Go."

Objective: to elicit and share memories of work experiences and to compare past and current occupations

Materials:
Pictures of workers in different occupations and work settings
Artifacts and pictures of work items (e.g., slide rule)
Written descriptions of obsolete occupations (e.g., movie theater usher)

Activities:
Sing-along using work-related songs
Pass around work-related objects and pictures of objects as you describe their function
Use job descriptions of obsolete occupations to elicit associations and naming (e.g., soda jerk, lamplighter); follow up with a discussion of factors that made the occupations obsolete
Generate a list of contemporary occupations that did not exist during the participants' childhood (e.g., fast-food workers)

Discussion starters:
"Describe the best/worst job you ever had."
"What did you admire/dislike about your boss?"
"How were you paid?"
"What was the first big-ticket item you bought with your earnings?"

Discussion expanders: Tell us about . . .
what your job responsibilities entailed.
your first promotion or pay raise.
the least/most time you worked at the same job.
what you would expect to be paid today for the work you did then.
the best advice you have for a young person who is entering the workforce.

---

depending on the abilities of the group members. The clinician does not lead the group but provides an atmosphere of support and guidance that enables group members to help each other. A specific sequence of activities for the procedural story task is provided in Table 8.4.

Commentary

For clinicians interested in learning more about CGT, see the text by Avent[8] and related education literature.[9–11]

PAINTING A PICTURE

The Complex Aphasia Rehabilitation Model (CARM) contains both individual and group treatment components.[12] Pachalska reports that

---

Making Mashed Potatoes

Nothing goes better with a pan of gravy than mashed potatoes. However, making mashed potatoes takes many steps. First, you must wash and scrub the potatoes. Once the potatoes are clean, you should use a vegetable peeler or knife and peel the potatoes. When the potatoes are peeled, you should place them in a pot, fill the pot with water, and add a little salt. The pot should be placed on the stove. Bring the water to a boil and cook the potatoes until they are tender. The potatoes are tender when a fork or a knife can be inserted in each one easily. When the potatoes are cooked, you will next drain the potatoes in a colander. While the potatoes are still warm, add butter and milk to the potatoes and mix them all together. Some people use a potato masher for this job but others prefer to use an electric mixer. Mix the potatoes, butter, and milk together into the desired consistency, add salt and pepper to taste. When the mashed potatoes are seasoned as you like them, it's time to serve them.

Key Word List

mashed potatoes, clean, peel, cook, stove, drain, butter, milk, mix, and salt

---

Figure 8.1
Sample of procedural story with key word list. (Reprinted with permission from J Avent. Manual of Cooperative Group Treatment for Aphasia. Boston: Butterworth–Heinemann, 1997.)

Table 8.4
Treatment sequence for cooperative group treatment.

---

1. Clinician reads story.
2. Clinician and patients review story and compile list of 8–10 key words and phrases.
3. Recaller practices telling the story. When cueing is needed, the facilitator provides specific cues. The clinician prompts as necessary.
4. Recaller practices telling the story in 1 minute.
5. Facilitator and clinician provide feedback (debrief) to the recaller to improve performance.

Source: Reprinted with permission from J Avent. Manual of Cooperative Group Treatment for Aphasia. Boston: Butterworth–Heinemann, 1997.

one of the most interesting activities for patients with aphasia participating in this holistic approach involves painting of a single picture
by the group.[13] This activity is facilitated by two clinicians, an artist
trained in occupational therapy, and a clinical aphasiologist. Groups
usually involve three or four persons and meet for 1 hour twice
weekly. The technique, according to Pachalska, gives the patient an
opportunity to restore a particular component of the language system,
painting. In this CARM activity, patients are able to use language in
context, participate in face-to-face conversations, and use multiple
channels to convey messages.

COMMENTARY

Detailed explanation of CARM is beyond the scope of this book. The
use of graphic abilities, such as painting and drawing, however, as
an output channel for expressively reduced aphasic patients should
not be overlooked. Some persons with aphasia convey more information through their drawings than through other channels.[14]
Although painting is wonderful, I am not sure that all clinicians have
the time to prepare and clean up after a painting session. Pencils,
chalk, or felt-tip pens might work as well. Group participants might
work together to draw a map of how to get to a certain section of
their city or to create a picture of a site that was familiar to all group
members (e.g., Statue of Liberty).

BARGAINING GAMES

As an extension of Promoting Aphasic Communicative Effectiveness
(PACE) therapy, Pulvermuller and Roth describe the bargaining
game.[15] Five illustrated cards are placed on a table between the patients
and the clinician. The cards depict activities that the participants can
take part in. Round 1 of the game involves bargaining as to which
activity the participants will select. The game sequence includes the
following speech acts: proposing, rejecting a proposal, and quoting
arguments for and against the proposal. For lower-level patients, specific linguistic forms can be practiced. For example, use of the modal
verb ("I would like to go for a swim.") can be trained. In the arguing
segment, complex sentences using words such as "if," "because,"
"since," and "for" can be used. The bargaining game can be played on
different levels of complexity. More severely involved patients may
require the pictures to be shown through the interaction and may need
to relate to the pictures by pointing. More advanced patients may need
to see the pictures only initially, or refer to the activities using action
verbs during the bargaining session.

Pulvermuller and Roth consider the bargaining game an extension of Davis and Wilcox's PACE therapy.[16, 17] Their paper on this subject does not target the use of this technique with groups per se, but it takes little imagination to think of how the bargaining game can be adapted to a group situation. Patients like to debate, argue, and do what they can to get their way. A great deal of discussion and interaction might come from a bargaining game that centered on where the group might go to have lunch together or what they might do on a specific planned outing.

DECISION MAKING

When someone becomes aphasic, he or she is not spared from making life's simple and complicated decisions. He or she still must decide whether to buy a new car, to rent or buy a house, or to have the house painted. Once a decision is made, he or she must implement a plan. Group meetings are excellent times to facilitate decision making and planning.

> Ms. Y. was a 71-year-old widow with moderate aphasia who attended a weekly aphasia group. She needed to have her house painted, but this type of task had always been handled by her deceased husband. Within the group, she and other participants worked together to plan how she could have her house painted. Issues of cost, quality, color, and scheduling were discussed. Group members with knowledge about painting houses visited her home to advise her on preparation, and whether all or a portion of the structure needed painting. Group members pooled their knowledge of reputable local house painters. On their recommendation, Ms. Y. solicited bids from three painters and obtained references from persons familiar with their work. These results were discussed in the group.

Ms. Y. was satisfied with her decision. The communicative value of this activity for the group was enormous.

Decision making and problem solving are an integral part of life. Group situations offer opportunities to discuss pros and cons of certain decisions and to do the problem solving needed to arrive at the best decision at the time. To make decision making a part of a group therapy program, the clinician should have an awareness of what is going on in the lives of group members.

COMMUNICATION SNAGS

Most persons with aphasia, regardless of its severity, worry about what will happen to them if they encounter a situation in which communication is important and they are likely to fail.[18, 19] For example, a frequently cited fear of many patients is that they will be perceived as drunk or mentally incompetent if they cannot communicate in an emergency. Others worry about how they will obtain and remember information important to their health when they visit their physician who is often on a tight schedule. Many aphasic persons wrestle with whether to inform their communication partners that they have had a stroke. Group treatment activities that teach patients how to handle these communication snags pay handsome dividends. They promote patient independence and self-esteem.

> Mr. J. was traveling home from New Zealand. Normally a fluent speaker with moderate word-finding problems, he found himself speechless when asked specific questions by a customs agent. Mr. J. and his group had worked on developing personalized emergency identification cards to use in such situations. Mr. J.'s card stated (1) that he had aphasia, a language problem, which caused him to have problems speaking in pressured situations, (2) that he had no problems understanding, (3) that the person should speak with him in a certain way, and (4) that someone could call his sister in case of an emergency. Once the agent saw this card, Mr. J. was moved through the line.

COMMENTARY

Several examples of how group treatment can be used to teach patients with aphasia how to deal with specific communication situations are provided in publications on group treatment of mild aphasia.[18, 19]

LOW-LEVEL PARTICIPATION

Occasionally, a patient in the group does not participate to the fullest extent. Reasons for the lack of participation vary. Some patients have problems initiating; others are just shy and reserved. Some patients believe they have nothing of importance to share. What the clinician does about this depends on many factors: the time needed to get the nonparticipant involved, patient motivation, and patient activity level. Sometimes, however, a concerted effort to give the patient an assignment outside the group can help.

Table 8.5
Sequence for planning a group activity: going bowling.

---

1. Select activities the group is interested in pursuing (e.g., bowling, fishing, going out to eat, going to a baseball game).
2. Establish a hierarchy of tasks that will lead the group to independently perform the selected activity (e.g., identify bowling alley, set up transportation, determine cost, reserve lanes, inquire about discounts for seniors, determine handicap access, get bowling shoes, select scorekeeper).
3. Rehearse communication strategies to be used in the activity in role-playing scenarios with group members and clinician. Assign responsibilities for the activity based on communicative abilities (e.g., scorekeeper).
4. Participate in the activity with the understanding that group members are responsible for all communication. They are allowed to enlist help from other group members but not from a spouse, caregiver, or clinician.
5. Participate in debriefing session at subsequent group meeting: (a) Identify successes of the activity; (b) note unexpected problems encountered; and (c) make suggestions for coping with problems in the future.

Source: Data from L Fox. Recreation Focused Treatment for Generalization of Language Skills in Aphasia Patients. Presented at the American Speech-Language-Hearing Association, Seattle, November 1990.

> Mr. R., a patient with severe Broca's aphasia, said little in group treatment. The clinician learned that Mr. R. and his wife had rented a motor home and were going to travel across the United States on a vacation. She asked Mr. R. to keep a diary about the trip by tape recording a few words and phrases at the end of each travel day. When Mr. R. returned, he was motivated to share his experiences. Moreover, knowing that he had been on a trip, group members were motivated to ask him questions about his travels. As a consequence, his participation level increased.

COMMENTARY

Reduced participation by one or more group members negatively affects the balance of a group. Good faith efforts to include those patients with low-level participation by giving them something specific to talk about may help.

PLANNING AN ACTIVITY

Field trips are an integral part of the education process. As former students, we remember these experiences vividly. For aphasic groups, planning a field trip or activity, engaging in the activity, and discussing it later offers many opportunities for working on communication skills. Table 8.5 provides a step-by-step outline for a planned activity—going bowling.[20] This activity is one of many possibilities. Consider going fishing, visiting a museum or library, taking a river boat excursion, seeing a movie or play, going to a baseball game, attending a concert, or engaging in some other pleasurable activity. Bargaining game strategies can be used in determining which activity the group will do. Activities break with routine and give the patient something to talk about with the group, family, and friends.

COMMENTARY

Group activities take place outside the treatment session. These activities typically take longer than the time scheduled for group meetings. This extra time, of course, may be problematic for the clinician. Consider including the spouses and caregivers of group members in the activity, but limit their direct participation in doing and communicating for group members. If the clinician cannot participate directly, participate vicariously by having group members and spouses share what happened at the outing at the next group meeting.

PREPARING A MEAL

Santo Pietro and Boczko use an activity they call the *breakfast club* to provide communicative opportunities for institutionalized patients with Alzheimer's disease.[21] If your facility has a kitchen, consider using this space for a group session where the objective would be to prepare a dish from a new recipe or prepare a simple meal. Preparing a meal offers a possibility for collaborative group work by rehabilitation team members (e.g., occupational therapy and speech-language pathology). It is an in-house activity rich in interactive communicative opportunities. The planning and organization of this type of activity might proceed similarly to that of planning a field trip. Group members will need to do some bargaining about what will be prepared in the kitchen, giving consideration to preparation and cleanup time. A list of ingredients needed for the recipe will need to be prepared, offering an opportunity to work on writing, spelling, and auditory memory skills. Kitchen implements needed to prepare the recipe should be identified and procured if not already available. Decisions should be made as to what ingredients are needed, in what amounts, at what cost, and where they are to be purchased. Roles should be assigned (e.g., buying the food, cooking the food, cleaning up, and setting the table). Following a recipe is also a good way to work on reading and sequencing skills.

COMMENTARY

Anyone who has tried to cook something for the first time realizes that cooking is a complex, highly communicative endeavor involving multiple processes. Keep what you do in the clinic very simple so that you can finish things on time. Allow plenty of time. People with aphasia move more slowly and require more time to do this task than do nonaphasic people.

COMPETITION TASKS

Competitiveness comes to us naturally. Group members enjoy friendly competition. Card games, charades, and board games are among the competitive games that can be used in a group situation that provide opportunities for working on cognitive communication skills as well. One game that appears to adapt well to group situations is 20 Questions. The 20 Questions task (20Q) is a verbal task that examines the patient's ability to ask questions to solve a problem. In this task, the patient views an array of pictures of common objects that are members of certain categories (e.g., food, transportation). The patient is instructed to ask yes/no questions to identify the object the examiner is thinking of by asking as few questions as possible. Better questions (e.g., Is it a fruit?) constrain the stimulus field and eliminate items from consideration regardless of the answer. Poor questions (e.g., Is it the apple?) reflect random guessing and have an immediate payoff for a yes answer but no payoff for a no answer. Narrowing questions (e.g., Is it a dessert?) further limit the choices after the category (e.g., food) has been identified. The number of pictures in the array can be adjusted in accordance with the severity of the patient's problem. Performance on the 20Q can be quantified along several dimensions. This task has been used in the assessment of the verbal performance of brain-injured persons by a number of investigators.[22–24]

COMMENTARY

20Q tasks are simple to create and highly adaptable to use in group situations. The 20Q paradigm can also be used with everyday problems (e.g., "John had to excuse himself from class at 10:00 AM. Why?") and situations (e.g., "What are the questions you need to ask when buying a car?") in addition to the picture format.

CONVERSATION PIECES

Occasionally, the group leader and the group itself will search for a topic of discussion. Lowrie and Nicholaus provide an extensive list of thought-provoking questions that would be stimulating in any group session.[25] In the "conversation piece," they ask questions such as, "If you could choose up to seven words to have on your epitaph, besides name and dates, what would the words say?" Another example is, "If you could avoid one household chore for the rest of your life, what chore would it be?"

COMMENTARY

Many of the questions in the conversation piece are unique. From an accountability standpoint, groups might respond to these questions more than once. If so, responses to questions might be compared across group sessions to see whether improvements were present in narratives, participatory levels of group members, turn taking, and other behaviors.

RESOURCES FOR GROUP
TREATMENT MATERIALS

The resources and materials for group treatment are abundant. Appendix 8.1 provides a list of resources for planning group treatment activities that may be useful. However, no substitution is available for creativity and innovation. I hope that clinicians interested in a long-term commitment to running an aphasia group will not limit themselves to commercially available materials and that they create materials and develop activities uniquely suited to their specific groups.

REFERENCES

1. Marshall RC. Case Studies in Aphasia Rehabilitation. Austin, TX: Pro-Ed, 1986.
2. Bollinger RL, Muson ND, Holland AL. A study of group communication intervention with chronically aphasic persons. Aphasiology 1993;7:301.
3. Jenkins TR, Knapp AC, Kelter AJ, Laird ME. Transdisciplinary Group Treatment: An Innovative Concept for Adults with Brain Injuries. Paper presented at the American Speech-Language-Hearing Association Convention, Boston, November 1997.
4. Harris JL. Reminiscence: a culturally and developmentally appropriate language intervention for older adults. Am J Speech-Lang Pathol 1997;6:19.
5. Butler RN. The life review: an interpretation of reminiscence in the aged. Psychiatry 1963;23:65.

6. Lubinski R, Masters MG. Special Populations, Special Settings: New and Expanding Frontiers. In R Lubinski, C Fratelli (eds), Professional Issues in Speech-Language Pathology and Audiology. San Diego: Singular, 1994;149.
7. Avent J. Group treatment in aphasia using cooperative learning methods. J Med Speech-Lang Pathol 1997;5:9.
8. Avent J. Manual of Cooperative Group Treatment for Aphasia. Boston: Butterworth–Heinemann, 1997.
9. Slavin RE. Cooperative Learning: Theory, Research, and Practice. Boston: Allyn & Bacon, 1995.
10. Larson CO, Cansereau DF. Cooperative learning in dyads. J Reading 1986;29:516.
11. Deutsch M. A theory of cooperation and competition. Hum Rel 1949;2:129.
12. Pachalska M. Group therapy for aphasia patients. Aphasiology 1991;5:541.
13. Pachalska M, Knapic H, Rogowski P, Perzanowski Z. Group Art Therapy Program and Functional Communication of Patients with Aphasia. In O Schindler, A Basso (eds), Aphasia Today: Proceedings of the First International Rehabilitation Congress, Florence, 1988;119.
14. Lyon J. Drawing: its value as a communicative aid for adults with aphasia. Aphasiology 1995;9:33.
15. Pulvermuller F, Roth VM. Communicative aphasia treatment as a further development of PACE therapy. Aphasiology 1991;5:39.
16. Davis GA. Pragmatics and Treatment. In R Chapey (ed), Language Intervention Strategies in Adult Aphasia (2nd ed). Baltimore: Williams & Wilkins, 1986;251.
17. Davis GA, Wilcox MJ. Adult Aphasia Rehabilitation: Applied Pragmatics. San Diego: College Hill Press, 1985;1.
18. Marshall RC. A Problem-Focused Group Treatment Program for Clients with Mild Aphasia. In R Elman (ed), Group Treatment for Aphasia: The Expert Clinician's Approach. Boston: Butterworth–Heinemann, 1999.
19. Marshall RC. Problem focused group treatment for clients with mild aphasia. Am J Speech-Lang Pathol 1993;2:31.
20. Fox L. Recreation Focused Treatment for Generalization of Language Skills in Aphasia Patients. Paper presented at the American Speech-Language-Hearing Association Convention, Seattle, November 1990.
21. Santo Pietro JM, Boczko F. The Breakfast Club and Related Programs. In BB Shadden, MA Toner (eds), Aging and Communication: For Clinicians by Clinicians. Austin, TX: Pro-Ed, 1997;117.
22. Marshall RC, Harvey S, Freed DB, Phillips DS. Question-Asking Strategies of Aphasic and Non–Brain-Damaged Adults. In M Lemme (ed), Clinical Aphasiology. Austin, TX: Pro-Ed, 1996;181.
23. Goldstein F, Levin HS. Question-asking strategies after severe closed head injury. Brain Cogn 1991;17:23.
24. Laine M, Butters N. A preliminary study of the problem-solving strategies of detoxified alcoholics. Drug Alcohol Depend 1982;10:235.
25. Lowrie P, Nicholaus B. The Conversation Piece. New York: Questmare Publishing, 1994.

Appendix 8.1

Sources for Materials

FROM GROUP MEMBERS

- Newspapers
- Newspaper articles (e.g., "Dear Abby")
- Magazine articles
- Printouts of stories or other information from the Internet
- Photo albums and journals
- Board games
- Old artifacts and memorabilia

FROM LIBRARY

- Old-time or classic films (e.g., newsreels, movies)
- Children's books
- Cookbooks
- Travel tapes (e.g., "Visit New Zealand")
- Craft books
- Books of short stories
- Magazines (e.g., *People, Sports Illustrated, Reader's Digest*)
- *Large Print Reader's Digest*
- Talking books (i.e., books on tape)

FROM COMMUNITY RESOURCES

- Posters, photographs of classic movie stars (from music stores)
- Travel brochures, maps (from travel agency)

- Atlases and maps (e.g., from the American Automobile Association)
- Restaurant menus (from different restaurants)

SELECTED COMMERCIAL SOURCES
OF MATERIALS

Bayles KA, Tomoeda CK. Pastimes. Tucson, AZ: Canyonlands, 1995.

Dikenjil AT, Kaye ME. Building Functional Social Skills: Group Activities for Adults. Tucson, AZ: Communication Skill Builders, 1988. Available from Communication Skill Builders, 3830 E. Bellevue, P.O. Box 42050, Tucson, AZ 85733.

Do You Remember When? Tucson, AZ: Communication Skill Builders, 1988. Available from Communication Skill Builders, 3830 E. Bellevue, P.O. Box 42050, Tucson, AZ 85733.

Hahn S, Klein ER. Focus on Function: Retraining for the Communicatively Impaired Client. Tucson, AZ: Communication Skill Builders, 1989. Available from Communication Skill Builders, 3830 E. Bellevue, P.O. Box 42050, Tucson, AZ 85733.

Lowrie P, Nicholaus B. The Conversation Piece. New York: Questmare Publishing, 1994;1.

Timeline. Remembering Work Life. Madison, WI: BiFokal Productions, 1997.

Zachman L, Barrett M, Huisingh R, et al. Tasks of Problem-Solving. A Real Life Approach to Thinking and Reasoning. East Moline, IL: LinguiSystems, 1992.

III

Documentation

9

Documentation in the Treatment Session

If group treatment truly improves the communication of persons with aphasia and over time reduces the psychosocial handicaps associated with aphasia, we must prove it.[1–3] Documentation, which takes many forms, provides this proof.[4–7] Documentation can involve numeric values associated with test scores, percentages correct, and rating scale values. It may focus on how tasks and issues addressed in treatment influence a patient's day-to-day functioning (e.g., talking on the telephone, ordering food in a restaurant). It may supply social validation data from unbiased observers about changes in the patient's behavior. The ultimate goal of documentation is always the same, whatever its form: to educate those who pay for aphasia treatment about how treatment helps the patient.[4]

The section on documentation of group treatment has three components. This chapter focuses on documenting what happens in the treatment session itself. Chapter 10 overviews communicative and psychosocial outcome measures that are useful in documenting the efficacy and the effectiveness of group treatment on a monthly basis. Chapter 11 deals with issues of social validation. No documentation strand is more or less important than any other. All strands collectively "paint a picture" of what treatment accomplishes.

THE TREATMENT SESSION

So much goes on within a group treatment session that the clinician may have difficulty keeping track of what is happening. The clinician has her or his hands full ensuring equal participation, deciding when to prompt and cue, providing clarification, keeping discussions on the topic, settling disputes, and so forth. Taking copious notes during a session is a challenge. Without taking notes, however, the clinician can easily forget what happened in the group session, impeding the accuracy of later documentation. The process of documentation begins with an account of what goes on in each treatment session. A useful paradigm is to think of how you can account for who said what, to whom, and how. This information, collected over a period of weeks, will allow the clinician to write required monthly progress reports for billing purposes.

Assistance from Another Person

Help for the clinician in session-to-session documentation is available from several sources. If a group is co-led, the roles of facilitator and recorder can be alternated from session to session. Speech-language pathology students in training may be able to take notes or collect other data during the session. These tasks could be assigned to a speech-language pathology assistant (SLP-A) working under the supervision of a speech-language pathologist who holds the certificate of clinical competence from the American Speech-Language-Hearing Association and has prerequisite experience in providing group treatment. These forms of assistance ensure that what goes on in the session will indeed be documented and free the group leader to direct the activities and actions of the group, thus maximizing stimulation for each participant. Notes taken during the session by any type of assistant (e.g., cofacilitator, student, or SLP-A) can be put into narrative form at a later time. Preparing the printed narrative can be a collaborative effort between the leader and the assistant.

Recording

An alternative to taking notes is to videotape some or all of the group sessions. A wall-mounted camera is needed to capture a wide-angle view of the entire group. Group members might need to sit in certain places to accomplish this feat. A sensitive microphone should be placed in a central location to pick up all that is said. In some organizations, group members may need to sign release forms to be videotaped.

More sophisticated and more expensive videotape setups are also available. These setups allow multiple angle views of the group members that facilitate capturing paralinguistic, nonverbal, and other aspects of communicative interactions. Recording all that happens in a group session on videotape comes at a price; someone has to review the tape. If the tape needs to be transcribed, it takes time. The more in-depth the analysis of the tape, the more time will be needed. One way to reduce the amount of time and work involved is to videotape

selected 15-minute segments of each group session. Another alternative is to record only a portion of group sessions each month (e.g., one
of four). If you are fortunate enough to have an audiovisual services
department in the workplace, you may be able persuade them to film
these recordings for you.

Boilerplate Forms

A simple boilerplate form can be created for session-by-session documentation purposes. It should contain the following information: date,
names of participants, group objectives, activities or tasks worked on,
ratings of behaviors exhibited during the session by group members,
and room for anecdotal comments by the clinician. A boilerplate is
strictly an in-house record of what occurs in a session. The clinician
uses these records to construct the monthly progress reports on specific group members. Boilerplate forms can be customized to fit any
group situation. Figure 9.1 is an example of a boilerplate form for a
group of four patients with moderately severe aphasia.

TRACKING FORMS

In some cases, session-to-session documentation can be accomplished
by using tracking forms or checklists. These instruments are useful in
noting the occurrence, type, and appropriateness of communicative,
pragmatic, and other behaviors of participants during the session.

Pragmatic Protocol

The pragmatic protocol[1] (Figure 9.2), although not specifically intended
for use in group sessions, is useful in charting the occurrence and
appropriateness of pragmatic behaviors of group participants when the
session or a portion of it is videotaped. In scoring the protocol, the
examiner notes the presence and appropriateness of 30 pragmatic parameters of language in three categories: verbal, paralinguistic, and nonverbal (see Figure 9.2). Designating a behavior as appropriate means
that it facilitates communicative interaction (e.g., an appropriate
request for repetition); behaviors judged to be inappropriate detract
from the communicative interchange and penalize the individual (e.g.,
asking for a repetition before the statement has been finished). One
way to use the pragmatic protocol is to focus on a single patient in the
group for a 15-minute period. During this time, the leader makes a spe-

---

Date: June 30, 1998

Group objectives: This group of four men with moderate aphasia meets for 1 hour each week. Objectives are (1) to reduce the psychosocial effects of aphasia and improve social, vocational, and recreational integration; (2) to provide a safe environment to discuss physical, psychological, and social consequences of aphasia; and (3) to provide clients sufficient space to develop initiative.

Members present: Joe R., Pete L., Ron G., Al C.

Topics: Joe's vacation plans; Pete having a foster child in the home; Ron's surgery; Al's recent seizure

Performance factors	Member				Comments
	JR	PL	RG	AC	
1. Participation level	3	4	3	1	Al depressed over seizure and medication change; low-level participation.
2. Adequacy of explanations	4	2	3	NA	Pete had a difficult time explaining the rules for having a foster child.
3. Listening	2	4	4	4	Good for all group members.
4. Interpersonal skills	2	3	3	NA	Joe needed reminders that others needed to talk.
5. Behavior	4	4	4	4	Ron used planning strategies developed in the group to ask his doctor relevant questions about his surgery. He and his wife feel much more optimistic.

Figure 9.1
Boilerplate documentation of group treatment session. (1 = poor; 2 = fair; 3 = good; 4 = normal; NA = not applicable.)

Communicative act	Appropriate	Inappropriate	Not observed
Verbal aspects			
A. Speech acts			
1. Speech act pair analysis			
2. Variety of speech acts			
B. Topic			
3. Selection			
4. Introduction			
5. Maintenance			
6. Change			
C. Turn taking			
7. Initiation			
8. Response			
9. Repair/revision			
10. Pause time			
11. Interruption/overlap			
12. Feedback to speakers			
13. Adjacency			
14. Contingency			
15. Quantity/conciseness			
D. Lexical selection/use			
16. Specificity/accuracy			
17. Cohesion			
E. Stylistic variations			
18. Varying communicative style			
F. Paralinguistic aspects			
19. Intelligibility			
20. Vocal intensity			
21. Prosody			
22. Vocal quality			
23. Fluency			
Nonverbal aspects			
G. Kenesics and proxemics			
24. Physical proximity			
25. Physical contacts			
26. Body posture			
27. Foot/leg and hand/arm			
28. Gestures			
29. Facial expression			
30. Gaze			

Figure 9.2
Items included on the pragmatic protocol. (Data from C Prutting, D Kirshner. A clinical appraisal of the pragmatic aspects of language. J Speech Hear Disord 1987;52[2]:105.)

cific effort to engage the group member in conversation or to get that person to interact with other group members. Different group members could be targeted for tracking with the protocol for each session.

The Profile of Communicative Appropriateness (PCA) identifies parameters of language that depend on both linguistic and extralinguistic context in a speaker's conversation.[2] The PCA is a more complex instrument than the pragmatic protocol, but it also can be adapted to record information from a group setting.

Process Evaluation Checklist

Loverso, Young-Charles, and Tonkovich use a process evaluation form to assess patients' roles within group settings.[3] This form specifies certain communication tasks, maintenance, and nonfunctional behaviors seen in the group setting. Task behaviors include evaluating, initiating, elaborating, summarizing, information giving, and information seeking. Maintenance behaviors include encouraging, harmonizing, gatekeeping, and standard setting and following. Nonfunctional behaviors, those that interfere with group processes, include blocking, self-directing, disrupting, and distorting. Table 9.1 provides a brief definition of each of these behaviors. Intertester reliability ratings of the presence of task, maintenance, and nonfunctional behaviors for three raters who observed two sessions of group treatment involving four patients were found to be within acceptable limits. The presence and occurrences of these behaviors should be charted for group members across the entire group session.

Activity Participation Checklist

When the group treatment session is activity-oriented, members' participation can also be summarized with a checklist. An example of a checklist that might be completed for each patient participating in a weekly group session is provided in Figure 9.3.[4] The form rates activity-related (e.g., attentiveness) and language-related (e.g., following the main idea) behaviors on a 5-point scale. It allows the clinician to obtain an estimate of the "level of participation" illustrated by a patient during the activity.

Erskine, Moody, and Rau developed a checklist similar to that shown in Figure 9.3 for use with a group of patients with global aphasia.[5] This form permits the examiner to rate communicative behaviors unique to patients with global aphasia (e.g., gaze, posture, facial expression, and use of variations in pitch, intensity, and duration) that are used during group activities. Ratings are made using a 5-point scale. Raters indicate,

Table 9.1
Task, maintenance, and nonfunctional behaviors included
in process evaluation form.

Task behaviors
    Evaluating: determining group difficulties and/or evaluating group progress
    Initiating: suggestion of ideas; new definition of problem
    Elaborating: clarifying; envisioning an idea if adopted
    Summarizing: restating ideas after discussion
    Information giving: offering facts or opinions; restating experiences
    Information seeking: asking for ideas; wanting feedback
Maintenance behaviors
    Encouraging: willing to hear others; supportive of the group
    Harmonizing: relieving dispute; compromising
    Gatekeeping: making sure all members are heard
    Standard setting: expressing standards for group after discussion
    Following: going along with group norms and discussions
Nonfunctional behaviors
    Blocking: arguing; rejecting ideas before they are heard
    Self-directing: hidden agendas; self-aggrandizement
    Disrupting: group clown; joker
    Distorting: distorting facts, ideas, or decisions

Source: Reprinted with permission from FL Loverso, H Young-Charles, J Tonkovich.
The Application of a Process Evaluation Form for Aphasic Individuals in a Small
Group Setting. In R Brookshire (ed), Clinical Aphasiology Conference Proceedings.
Minneapolis: BRK, 1982;10.

when possible, how the information was conveyed: with a gesture, verbal language (words), or by a vocal production other than a word.

Pragmatics and Communication Summary Sheet

Fox uses a checklist with her recreation-focused group for patients with severe aphasia. This tool facilitates tracking of pragmatic and communication behaviors believed to be important in charting the progress of group members.[6] Communication behaviors used by patients in the group are tallied throughout the session. Other behaviors are rated on a 7-point scale. This checklist is shown in Table 9.2.

Perceptions of Interactional Competence

Groups involve interaction among the participants, the group leader, and other persons (e.g., guests or speakers). Garrett and Sittner use a

Activity-related behavior	Never 1	Poor 2	Fair 3	Good 4	Normal 5
1. Did the patient attend to the activity?	—	—	—	—	—
2. Was his/her behavior appropriate to the task?	—	—	—	—	—
3. Did the patient participate in the activity independently?	—	—	—	—	—
4. Did the patient follow the suggestions that were given?	—	—	—	—	—
5. Did the patient generate ideas for the future activities?	—	—	—	—	—
Language-related activity					
1. Did the patient attend to what others said?	—	—	—	—	—
2. Did the patient follow the main ideas of others?	—	—	—	—	—
3. Did the patient initiate communication without clinician direction?	—	—	—	—	—
4. Were the patient's responses appropriate?	—	—	—	—	—
5. Did the patient communicate ideas clearly?	—	—	—	—	—

Patient's name: _____ Mean score: _____

Figure 9.3
Checklist of activity and language-related behaviors. (Information from J Aten. A Round Table Discussion on Group Treatment. In R Brookshire [ed], Clinical Aphasiology Conference Proceedings. Minneapolis: BRK, 1981;142.)

Table 9.2
Pragmatics and communication progress summary sheet.

Communication behaviors observed
  1. Topic initiation/changes
  2. Requests for information
  3. Comments on a topic
  4. Interjected comments on own communication abilities
  5. Responses to an elicitation
  6. Feedback to another speaker/reiteration of another's comment
  7. Repairs or revisions after a request for an explanation
  8. Interruptions
  9. Ambiguous or unintelligible utterances
Interactive behaviors (rate 1–7; 7 = good/always; 1 = poor/never)
  1. Introducing new topics
  2. Clear presentation of information
  3. Attending behavior
  4. Use of auxiliary modes of expression when needed

Source: Data from L Fox. Recreation Focused Treatment for Generalization of Language Skills in Aphasic Patients. Presented at the American Speech-Language-Hearing Association, Seattle, November 1990.

questionnaire similar to that shown in Figure 9.4 to rate "interactional competence." Their 7-point rating scale has been used successfully in group treatment situations.[7] The authors report that untrained observers can perform perceptual ratings of interactional competence of aphasic patients in a group situation with a high degree of reliability and that higher ratings are typically assigned to patients with mild aphasia and vice versa. This scale offers a very simple and rapid means of documenting individual levels of participation in group settings. More measures like that in Figure 9.4 are needed, given the time constraints of present day speech-language pathologists.

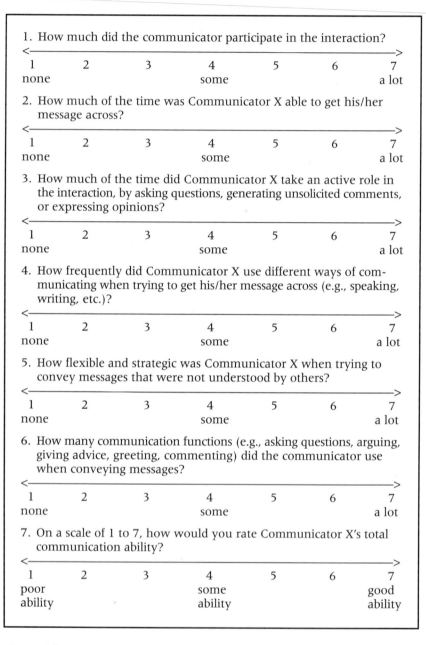

1. How much did the communicator participate in the interaction?

```
<———————————————————————————————————————————>
1        2        3        4        5        6        7
none                      some                      a lot
```

2. How much of the time was Communicator X able to get his/her message across?

```
<———————————————————————————————————————————>
1        2        3        4        5        6        7
none                      some                      a lot
```

3. How much of the time did Communicator X take an active role in the interaction, by asking questions, generating unsolicited comments, or expressing opinions?

```
<———————————————————————————————————————————>
1        2        3        4        5        6        7
none                      some                      a lot
```

4. How frequently did Communicator X use different ways of communicating when trying to get his/her message across (e.g., speaking, writing, etc.)?

```
<———————————————————————————————————————————>
1        2        3        4        5        6        7
none                      some                      a lot
```

5. How flexible and strategic was Communicator X when trying to convey messages that were not understood by others?

```
<———————————————————————————————————————————>
1        2        3        4        5        6        7
none                      some                      a lot
```

6. How many communication functions (e.g., asking questions, arguing, giving advice, greeting, commenting) did the communicator use when conveying messages?

```
<———————————————————————————————————————————>
1        2        3        4        5        6        7
none                      some                      a lot
```

7. On a scale of 1 to 7, how would you rate Communicator X's total communication ability?

```
<———————————————————————————————————————————>
1        2        3        4        5        6        7
poor                      some                      good
ability                   ability                   ability
```

Figure 9.4

Questionnaire for rating interactional competence of aphasic patients in a group setting. (Data from K Garrett, M Sittner. Perceptions of Interactional Competence of Persons with Aphasia. Paper presented at American Speech-Language-Hearing Association, Orlando, FL, December 1996.)

REFERENCES

1. Prutting C, Kirshner D. A clinical appraisal of the pragmatic aspects of language. J Speech Hear Disord 1987;52(2):105.
2. Penn C. The profiling of syntax and pragmatics in aphasia. Clin Ling Phon 1988;2(3):179.
3. Loverso FL, Young-Charles H, Tonkovich J. The Application of a Process Evaluation Form for Aphasic Individuals in a Small Group Setting. In R Brookshire (ed), Clinical Aphasiology Conference Proceedings. Minneapolis: BRK, 1982;10.
4. Aten J. A Round Table Discussion on Group Treatment. In R Brookshire (ed), Clinical Aphasiology Conference Proceedings. Minneapolis: BRK, 1981;142.
5. Erskine B, Moody CS, Rau MT. Group Treatment for Globally Aphasic Individuals. Paper presented at the Oregon and Washington Speech and Hearing Association, Seattle, October 1987.
6. Fox L. Recreation Focused Treatment for Generalization of Language Skills in Aphasic Patients. Paper presented at the American Speech-Language-Hearing Association Convention, Seattle, November 1990.
7. Garrett K, Sittner M. Perceptions of the Interactional Competence of Persons with Aphasia. Paper presented at the American Speech-Language-Hearing Association Convention, Orlando, December 1995.

10

Monthly Documentation

The standard procedure for treatment recertification is a monthly report of patient progress. The report is sent to a reviewer who may be a nurse, physician, speech-language pathologist, related professional (e.g., physical therapist), or screening clerk. On the basis of the report's content, a determination about the necessity of continuing treatment will be made. Monthly reports are standard for patients seen for individual treatment for aphasia. A standard for the frequency of reports for patients receiving group treatment has not been established. Unless a different standard is implemented for groups, the frequency with which clinicians report results of group treatment will likely be on a monthly basis as well. The data from the weekly sessions (see Chapter 9) is used to construct monthly treatment summaries. These data are supplemented by other measures that are largely objective. The clinician has a number of options in selecting documentation measures.

SELECTING THE DOCUMENTATION TOOL

Nothing is more important for good documentation than selecting the right instrument to measure the effects of group or any other treatment.[1] The instrument the clinician chooses should match very closely what he or she is attempting to accomplish in therapy. For example, a goal of some aphasia groups is to encourage patients to communicate their thoughts in any way possible. This technique suggests that total communication strategies—combining speaking, writing, drawing, gesturing, and pointing—are emphasized.[2] When using total communication strategies, a documentation tactic that only assesses how well the patient talks will not reflect how the patient is improving in group treatment. A verbally oriented measure will (1) not show how the patient uses other modes of communication and (2) misrepresent what treatment is attempting to accomplish.

Selecting the right instrument, rating scale, or other measure to document progress for each individual in a group depends on several factors, including (1) group treatment goals and objectives, (2) time available for measurement and documentation, (3) frequency and duration of group treatment, (4) examiner skill, and (5) requirements for documentation imposed on the clinician by the agency to which the report will be sent. In this section, I present some methods for objective documentation of progress for individual patients seen in groups. These methods include (1) periodic administration of standardized tests, (2) measures for quantifying verbal output, (3) communication effectiveness ratings, and (4) indices of well-being, life satisfaction, and other psychosocial measures.

STANDARDIZED TESTS

The standardized assessment instruments used most often in aphasia assessment are the Western Aphasia Battery (WAB),[3] Porch Index of Communicative Ability (PICA),[4] Boston Diagnostic Aphasia Examination (BDAE),[5] and the Minnesota Test for Differential Diagnosis of Aphasia (MTDDA).[6] All take at least 1 hour to complete; most take much longer. A clinician with a four-patient group who is required to submit a monthly progress report for each patient would therefore spend a minimum of 4 hours in test administration each month. If the group only meets weekly, testing time exceeds that spent in treatment. Although advantageous from many standpoints, measuring a patient's progress in group treatment with a standardized examination is not realistic. It takes too much time. The MTDDA and the PICA have shortened forms that yield equivalent overall scores to their longer versions.[7-9] The short forms are options for the clinician who wants to use or may be required to measure progress with a standardized measure by the health care agency.

The use of standardized test batteries as a primary means of documenting group treatment results poses other dilemmas. One is that these batteries are far more sensitive to an aphasic person's linguistic disabilities than to his or her functional and psychosocial disabilities. The WAB, PICA, MTDDA, and BDAE provide information about severity of aphasia, where performance breaks down in each modality, and a patient's linguistic strengths and weaknesses. They tell us less about how the patient communicates in naturalistic settings or how aphasia handicaps day-to-day functioning. A second problem is that standardized tests may not be sensitive enough to capture changes made in treatment by some group patients. This lack of sensitivity may particularly be the case when group participants are more chronic and therefore change less over time than do patients whose strokes are of more recent onset.

A strong case can be made for using a standardized test in monthly documentation in those cases when the aphasic individual begins group treatment within the first year postonset and treatment terminates within that first year. In such cases, the issue of sensitivity would be less important.

VERBAL OUTCOME MEASURES

When groups emphasize discussion and problem solving, improving narrative expression, maintaining a topic, and other expressive skills, change over time should be quantified with a verbal measure.[10–12] Several options exist, but again the clinician should select a verbal outcome measure that best fits his or her needs and work situation. For example, the amount of time needed to administer the verbal measure, transcribe, score the patient's utterances, and write up the results for the reviewer should be considered. The clinician must also consider whether the measure selected can graphically display change over time. Consider also whether using a particular verbal measure will require scheduling separate appointments for individual group members to undergo these verbal assessments, or whether the measure can be done by taking a few minutes at the conclusion of a weekly group session. The verbal outcome measures discussed in this section are not an all-inclusive list; they were selected to reflect some of the many options available.

Cookie Theft Narrative

Asking the patient to describe the cookie theft picture from the BDAE is a simple, objective way of quantifying connected speech samples of patients with aphasia. The patient is asked, "Tell me everything you see happening in this picture." The clinician audiotapes the narrative, transcribes the sample, and times the length of the sample in seconds with a stopwatch. Yorkston and Beukelman provide scoring guidelines for the procedure.[13] The connected sample is scored according to the amount of information conveyed (number of content units), the amount of information conveyed over time (number of content units per minute), and the speaking rate (and number of syllables per minute). Table 10.1 illustrates the use of this measure for a connected speech sample from a patient with anomic aphasia.

Table 10.1
Transcription of a connected speech sample describing the cookie theft picture from the Boston Diagnostic Aphasia Examination by a patient who developed an anomic aphasia secondary to viral encephalitis.

Description: "All right. The wuh, the *wife*, the *woman's doing* some *dishes*. She's *paying no attention*. The *water's running*. And it's going *all over the floor*. And her *children are*—*robbing* the *cookie jar*. And also, the *chair's* going to *fall over*. And one of them is going to *get hurt*, probably."
Time: 120 seconds
Number of syllables: 70
Number of content units*: 20
Rate: 102 syllables per minute (120/70 × 60)
Content units per minute: 10 content units per minute (120/20 × 60)

---

*Content units are in italics.

Linguistic Communication Measure

The Linguistic Communication Measure (LCM) also focuses on clinically relevant dimensions of aphasic narrative speaking performance.[14] It is similar to the cookie theft procedure in that it also measures the amount of information conveyed in content units. The LCM is also used for the cookie theft picture from the BDAE, but it can be used with other stimuli as well (e.g., pictures and narratives). Two additional components of the LCM are the indices of lexical efficiency and grammatic support. The former assesses the proportion of noninformative words or "emptiness of speech" and is helpful when a patient has anomic deficits. The latter reflects the number of supporting words and grammatic morphemes for the content units and is helpful when the patient has syntactic difficulties.

Correct Information Unit Analysis

A rule-based scoring system for evaluating the informativeness and efficiency of connected speech samples of persons with aphasia, the correct information unit (CIU) analysis can be used with a variety of elicitation stimuli. Stimuli used with the CIU include the WAB picnic scene, the cookie theft picture, two requests for personal information (e.g., "Tell me what you do on Sundays," "Tell me where you live and describe it to me."), two procedural discourse tasks (e.g., "Tell me how you go about doing the dishes by hand," "Tell me how you go about writing and sending a letter."), as well as two 6-picture sequences and two single pictures developed by the CIU authors.[15]

Two advantages of the CIU system are its explicit rule-based scoring system that tells the clinician what words should and should not be included in the analysis and its inclusion of a variety of elicitation stimuli. Nicholas and Brookshire found that all CIU elicitation stimuli were capable of measuring informativeness and efficiency of connected speech samples and that performance of aphasic subjects over time was relatively stable. This suggests that these stimuli, which are relatively easily administered, can be used to measure changes in connected speech over time.

Everyday Language Test

The Amsterdam-Nijmegen Everyday Language Test (ANELT) is another verbally oriented measure that assesses the level of verbal communication ability of an aphasic patient.[16] Two parallel versions of the test have been developed. Test items are based on scenarios of familiar daily life situations. For example, the examiner says, "You have an appointment with the doctor. Something else has come up. You call the doctor, and what do you say?" Responses to ANELT test items shown in Table 10.2 are rated on two scales. Scale A, understandability, reflects the content of the message to be communicated irrespective of its linguistic form. Scale B, intelligibility, relates to the perception of the message independent of its content or meaning. Scale ratings of understandability and intelligibility reflect five levels of ability: (1) not at all, (2) a little, (3) medium, (4) reasonable, and (5) good. A patient can have different ratings on the two scales. For example, if a patient responded, "Hi, Doctor um, um, oh forget it. Nuts!" his or her response would be rated high for intelligibility because it was clear, but low for understandability because the content of the message was not communicated. ANELT scenarios parallel those that might occur in the day-to-day life of the patient. Some reviewers might consider improvement over time in responding to these situations more representative of patient progress than improved descriptions of other stimuli.

Reporter's Test

The Reporter's Test is described as a sensitive measure to detect expressive disturbances of aphasic patients.[17] Essentially, this test is an expressive version of part V of the Token Test.[18] The patient's task is to describe verbally the examiner's manipulation of two types of tokens (circles and squares) of five colors (blue, red, white, green, yellow). If the examiner

Table 10.2
The Amsterdam-Nijmegen Everyday Language Test items.

---

1. You are now at the dry cleaners. You have come to pick this up and you get it back like this. [Present shirt with scorch mark.] What do you say?
2. The kids on the street are playing football in your yard. You have asked them before not to do that. You go outside and speak to the kids. What do you say?
3. You go to a store and want to buy a television. I am the salesperson here. "Can I help you?"
4. You go to the shoemaker with this shoe. [Present shoe.] There is a lot wrong with this shoe, but for some reason you want him to repair only one thing. You may choose what. What do you say?
5. You have an appointment with the doctor. Something else has come up. You call the doctor's office, and what do you say?
6. You are in the drug store and this [present glove] is lying on the floor. What do you say?
7. You see your neighbor walking by. You want to ask him or her to come to visit some time. What do you say?
8. Your neighbor's dog barks all day long. You are really tired of it. You want to talk to him about it. What do you say?
9. You have just moved next door to me. You would like to meet me. You ring my doorbell and say . . .
10. You are at the florist. You want to have a bouquet of flowers delivered to a friend. I am the salesperson. What do you say?

Source: Reprinted with permission from L Blomert, ML Kean, C Koster, J Schokker. Amsterdam-Nijmegen Everyday Language Test: construction, reliability, and validity. Aphasiology 1994;8:381.

places the yellow square on top of the green circle, the correct response would be, "You put the yellow square on top of the green circle." The patient's responses are recorded. The test is scored by playing the responses for a naive listener, who then "performs" the actions described by the patient. In a plus-minus scoring format, the response, "You put the yellow square on top of the green square" receives no points, but in a weighted system it receives four of five points. The patient is only penalized for use of the word "square" in lieu of circle.

Explanation

Explanations (e.g., "Tell me what you did today," "How do you play dominos?") and procedural discourse tasks (e.g., "Tell me the steps involved in making a pot of tea.") can be used to assess language skills of patients with aphasia and those with cognitive-communicative problems after traumatic brain injury (TBI). McDonald and Pearce described

Table 10.3
Rating scale for scoring of summarization task.

6	Normal performance. Good general summary and no irrelevancies.
5	Good general summary. Sounds almost normal but not quite.
4	Produces 5–6 specific memories with or without irrelevancies.
3	Produces 3–4 specific memories with or without irrelevancies.
2	Produces 1–2 specific memories with or without irrelevancies.
1	No specific memories; all irrelevancies.
0	No performance.

a procedure called "The Dice Game," in which the patient explains how to play dice to a naive listener.[19] The explanation is taped, orthographically transcribed, and the content quantified. This procedure is helpful in determining the distribution of essential and nonessential comments in the patient's explanations. The clinician need not be confined to an explanation of how to play dice. It is applicable to any board game (e.g., dominos, checkers, blackjack).

Summarization

Sometimes, treatment within a group situation seeks to help a patient be more "to the point" in communication. Summarization tasks are often used for this purpose. These tasks require a patient to listen or, preferably, read a passage and decide what is and is not important to include in a summary. Length of the reading passage can be adjusted according to the severity of the patient's aphasia. Rating procedures can be used to quantify the adequacy of the summary. Although no specific rating scales have been published for the purposes of rating summarizations per se, Table 10.3 provides an example of a scale for rating the adequacy of a summarization by a patient using a scoring system from the MTDDA quicksand story.[6] Summarization tasks as a means of documenting progress have been found to be useful with higher level aphasic, TBI, demented, and right hemisphere damaged patients.[20]

COMMUNICATIVE EFFICIENCY

Some patients with aphasia have assessment profiles that suggest they will not become verbal communicators. For these patients, treatment of the verbal modality may be limited to working on a few key words.

The goal of treatment for such patients is to promote communicating in whatever way possible. These expressively reduced aphasic (ERA) patients combine writing, drawing, gesturing, and pointing with their limited verbalizations to get their points across.[21] They may use or be taught to use facial expression, vocal intonations, and other paralinguistic cues to supplement their limited expression. Simple augmentative communication devices such as communication boards and written choice communication may be appropriate for these patients.[22, 23] Documentation may involve use of an overall measure of communicative efficiency or a task-specific measure.

OVERALL MEASURES OF COMMUNICATIVE EFFICIENCY

Overall communicative efficiency can be measured directly or indirectly. Direct measures require actually "doing something with a patient." Indirect measures involve rating communicative efficiency on the basis of what is known about a patient or what is observed in a communicative interaction. Three instruments that might be used by a clinician to measure group treatment progress for an ERA patient are reviewed in this section. One is a standardized test. Two others are rating scales that allow the clinician to rate a patient's functional adequacy in communication in a variety of situations based on knowledge about the patient. Not included in this section is information on the Functional Independence Measure (FIM), because it is more applicable to patients seen in more acute settings.[24]

Communicative Abilities of Daily Living

The CADL is a direct measure of communicative efficiency.[25] It is the only standardized aphasia test that gives a patient credit for getting a message across in any way possible. Responses to CADL items are scored on a 3-point scale. Successful attempts are scored as 2; "in the ballpark" efforts are scored 1; communication failures are scored 0. The 68 CADL items reflect communicative interactions that the patient is likely to encounter in daily life (e.g., reporting for a doctor's appointment). The clinician and patient role play each scenario in a context using props included in the test kit. The CADL is normed on aphasic and normal adults in both institutionalized and noninstitutionalized settings. CADL scores correlate highly with PICA scores. The CADL is a wonderful test to use with an ERA patient. Using the CADL as a means to document progress made by an ERA patient in group treat-

Table 10.4
Items included in the Communicative Effectiveness Index.

Item	Situation
1	Getting someone's attention
2	Getting involved in group conversations about him or her
3	Giving yes/no answers appropriately
4	Communicating his or her emotions
5	Indicating that he or she understands what is being said to him or her
6	Having coffee-time visits and conversations with friends and neighbors
7	Having a one-to-one conversation with you
8	Saying the name of someone whose face is in front of him or her
9	Communicating physical needs such as aches and pains
10	Having a spontaneous conversation
11	Responding to or communicating anything (including yes/no answers without words)
12	Starting a conversation with people who are not close family
13	Understanding writing
14	Being a part of a conversation when it is fast and a number of people are present
15	Participating in a conversation with strangers
16	Describing or discussing something at length

Source: Reprinted with permission from J Lomas, L Pickard, S Bester, et al. The Communicative Effectiveness Index: development and psychometric evaluation of a functional communication measure for adult aphasia. J Speech Hear Dis 1989;54:113.

ment poses problems with respect to administration time similar to those posed by other standardized tests.

Communicative Effectiveness Index

The CETI is a rating scale for estimating aphasic persons' communicative ability in specific communicative situations.[26] These situations fall into four categories: basic needs, life skills, social needs, and health threats. Table 10.4 shows the items included in the CETI. These items were generated from focus group meetings involving stroke patients and their spouses. The examiner rates each of the items on a 100-mm visual analog scale. A numeric value (1–100) is assigned to each item measured. Values of the 16 items are summed and averaged to yield an overall CETI index.

American Speech-Language-Hearing Association Functional Assessment of Communication Skills for Adults

The American Speech-Language-Hearing Association Functional Assessment of Communication Skills for Adults (ASHA-FACS) rates a patient's communicative adequacy in four domains: social communication; communication of basic needs; daily planning; and reading, writing, and number concepts.[27] Ratings are made using a 7-point scale of independence similar to that of the FIM, which is used in more acute settings.[27] An ASHA-FACS rating of 7 indicates that the patient performs the function with no assistance; a rating of 1 indicates that the patient cannot perform the task even with maximal assistance. Overall performance in each of the ASHA-FACS domains is also rated on dimensions of adequacy, promptness, appropriateness, and sharing of communicative burden. Table 10.5 summarizes the assessment domains of the ASHA-FACS.

Functional Communication Profile

The Functional Communication Profile (FCP) is the first measure to be used extensively in evaluation of aphasic patients' functional communication skills.[28] FCP performance is based on an interview with a patient after which the clinician rates the patient on five categories of communication behavior: movement, speaking, understanding, reading, and other. Each category contains communication behaviors regarded as representative of those occurring in everyday life (e.g., recognition of family names). Behaviors are rated on a 9-point scale in which the patient's present ability is rated in relation to his or her premorbid ability.

The FCP, as a single measure to document the effects of group treatment, poses some problems if the clinician must conduct a separate interview for each group patient. It may be possible to teach a significant other to perform an FCP rating on a monthly basis, however, providing they are willing to do so and the time for training is available. The FCP has also been revised for use in the United Kingdom.[29] The revised version measures communication functions and modalities used for greeting, acknowledging, responding, requesting, and initiating. The examiner rates a patient's ability on a 5-point effectiveness scale.

Functional Skills Survey

Payne has developed another rating scale, the Communication Profile: A Functional Skills Survey.[30] This rating scale is a patient self-reporting or caregiver-reporting measure that contains 26 items related to every-

Table 10.5

Assessment domains for the American Speech-Language-Hearing Association Functional Assessment of Communication Skills for Adults.

Social Communication/ Writing	Basic Needs	Daily Planning	Reading/Number Concepts
Uses names of familiar people	Recognizes familiar faces/voices	Tells time	Understands environmental signs
Expresses agreement/ disagreement	Makes strong likes/dislikes known	Dials phone numbers	Uses reference materials
Explains how to do something	Expresses feelings	Keeps appointments	Follows written directions
Participates in phone conversations	Makes needs/ wants known	Uses a calendar	Understands printed material
Answers yes/no questions	Responds in an emergency	Follows a map	Prints/writes/types name
Follows directions			Completes forms
Understands facial expression/tone of voice			Makes short lists
Understands nonliteral meaning and intent			Writes messages
Understands conversation in noisy surroundings			Understands signs with numbers
Understands television and radio			Makes money transactions
Participates in conversations			Understands units of measurement
Recognizes/ corrects errors			

Source: Reprinted with permission from American Speech-Language-Hearing Association. Functional Assessment of Communication Skills for Adults. Rockville, MD: American Speech-Language-Hearing Association, 1994.

day situations involving understanding, reading, speaking, and writing. Ratings are made using a 5-point scale that focuses on the *importance* of the skill. Importance is a key concept because it relates to the centrality of a skill in a patient's life. The Functional Skills Survey was developed as a tool that would, in the hands of an examiner, be sensitive to cultural, lifestyle, employment, and income differences, features not typically accounted for in other measures.

Speech Questionnaire

Lincoln's Speech Questionnaire includes 19 questions grouped into two areas, speech and understanding.[31] An example of a question in the speech section is, "Does he say any single words spontaneously (without help from you)?" An example of a question from the understanding section is, "Does he understand rapid conversation with more than one person?" The examiner rates the aforementioned types of questions using a Guttman scaling technique: often, sometimes, rarely, and never. This tool appears relatively simple to use and could easily be administered by persons other than the treating clinician on a monthly basis.

TASK-SPECIFIC MEASURES OF INFORMATION EXCHANGE

The clinician may use task-specific measures to quantify features of an ERA patient's communicative efficiency in the group. These features include (1) accuracy of message exchange, (2) speed of message exchange, and (3) degree of communicative burden assumed by the conversational partner. The clinician may also want to determine whether the modalities (e.g., drawing, pointing, and writing), compensatory efforts, and augmentative strategies used by a patient in message exchanges reflects what is being stressed in the group treatment sessions. The ideal way to use task-specific measures in the documentation process is to conduct a rating each week. Weekly ratings can then be used to determine improvement over time. This information is used in constructing monthly reports.

Message Exchange Task

Fawcus and Fawcus give patients in their aphasia program a message to convey to the caregiver on returning home.[32] The message is presented verbally to the patient; precautions are taken to ensure that the patient understands and can retain it long enough to convey it to

---

Patient name: _____ **Date:** _____

Message: <u>No therapy</u> on <u>August 27</u>. <u>Susan</u> has to <u>go to Miami</u> for her sister's wedding.

Under each word or idea conveyed, please indicate whether it was put across by

Writing (W)

Drawing (D)

Gesture (G)

Pointing (P)

Speaking (S)

A message may be put across in several different ways. For example,

The Red Sox lost the game on a ninth inning home run.
    W   G   G   D   G

Approximately how much time did it take to convey the message?

Less than 2 minutes _____ 2–5 minutes _____ Longer _____
Gave up _____

Figure 10.1
Example of a message exchange form. (Adapted from M Fawcus, R Fawcus. Information transfer in four cases of articulatory apraxia. Aphasiology 1990;4:207.)

the caregiver. The caregiver fills out a form similar to that provided in Figure 10.1. This information allows the clinician to assess (1) accuracy of message conveyance and (2) those specific modalities used by the patient to convey the message. To use this procedure as a documentation tool, the clinician can give the patient a message at the end of the group session each week. Improvement in message accuracy and use of communication modalities stressed in treatment can be measured over time.

Barrier Tasks

Barrier tasks are interactional: The patient sits on one side of the barrier; the partner sits on the other side. The patient directs the actions of the partner in performing a specific task such as arranging a room of dollhouse furniture in a specific way or drawing a crude plan of his or her home. A useful spin-off of the barrier task that does not require an actual

Rating of Communicative Efficiency

Communicative efficiency is defined as the "completeness, clarity, and speed with which the client conveys information in the exchange." Using the scale below, place an "X" between the two anchor points on the line provided.

No attempt to provide
any information

Complete
information

Rating of Communicative Burden

Communicative burden is defined as "the degree to which the partner needs to use inference, to question, and to guess in order to verify the accuracy of a message." Using the scale below, place an "X" between the two anchor points on the line provided.

Partner assumes
no communicative
burden

Partner assumes
all communicative
burden

Figure 10.2

Visual analog scales for rating communicative efficiency and communicative burden. (Data from RC Marshall, DB Freed, DS Phillips. Communicative efficiency in severe aphasia. Aphasiology 1997;11:373.)

barrier structure, is to have the patient use a city map to direct the partner to find his or her home or to find the location of a favorite restaurant.

Yorkston, Beukelman, and Flowers use a descriptive scale to rate accuracy and efficiency of message exchange: 4 = complete information, 3 = partially complete information, 2 = some relevant information, 1 = no relevant information, 0 = no attempt.[33] Visual analog rating scales similar to that shown in the upper portion of Figure 10.2 can also be used for rating accuracy and efficiency of message exchanges.[34] The scales should be 100 mm in length and have clearly defined anchor points that permit the clinician to convert a rating into a numeric value.

Communicative Burden

At times, knowing the degree of communicative burden assumed by the patient and his or her conversational partners may be helpful.

Linebaugh and colleagues view communicative burden as the portion of responsibility each participant in a conversation must bear to ensure the adequate transfer of information.[35] Communicative burden can be rated using a visual analog scale similar to that shown in the lower portion of Figure 10.2.

Speed of Message Exchange

A final objective measure, alluded to in all task-specific measures discussed previously, is speed of message exchange. When a patient with aphasia conveys messages faster from week to week, it may have the effect of reducing communicative burden on partners and increasing message accuracy. The increased speed may suggest that the patient is improving. Speed of message exchange can be measured with a handheld stopwatch in communicative turns during the treatment session. Measuring the speed of message exchange seems particularly easy when the sessions are recorded on videotape, and a person can be trained to do the timing.

PSYCHOSOCIAL OUTCOME MEASURES

The psychosocial and psychobehavioral issues that arise after a stroke are numerous and complex.[36, 37] A partial list includes depression, anxiety, mood alterations, sexual dysfunction, sleep disorders, loss of friends, marital difficulties, caregiver burnout, fear of another stroke, altered emotions, and other adjustment disorders. Depression scales, indices of well-being and general health, and other quality-of-life measures have been used extensively in the medical and social sciences. These measures are not discussed extensively here for two reasons: (1) Space to cover this topic is not sufficient, and (2) persons with aphasia who come to group treatment are more often chronic than acute. Their interests and those of their families relate to issues such as going out to dinner again, taking a trip, and talking with their children or grandchildren on the telephone. These and other personal concerns epitomize Lyon's plea for therapy to address the need of persons with aphasia to be able to "participate in life."[38, 39] For many patients, this need overrides improving scores on an aphasia test or using strategies taught by the clinician in treatment.[40] The psychosocial outcome measures discussed herein are restricted to those used by clinicians with aphasic patients. Information in Chapter 11 on social validation of group treatment outcomes also has relevance to the material presented in this chapter.

Mood Scales

Stern and coworkers developed a set of visual analog mood scales that provide brief, valid measures of internal mood states of brain-injured patients.[41] These scales are used with stroke and other neurologically impaired patients in rehabilitation settings. The mood scales use a 100-mm vertical line with brief descriptors (e.g., happy, sad) and simple pictures expressing the mood evaluated. For example, a "smiling face" would be connected to a "sad face" by a 100-mm vertical or horizontal line. The patient places a mark ("X") on the line, and the value is converted into a numerical equivalent. To assess moods of more impaired patients who might not be able to follow directions for completing a visual analog scale, the clinician can use index cards with simple terms and allow the patient to say or point to the card describing his or her mood. For example, if asking about anger, the patient can be shown four cards with the descriptive terms "very angry," "angry," "calm," and "very calm."

Psychological Well-Being Scale

Ryff uses a 14-item questionnaire to measure six dimensions of psychological well-being: self-acceptance, autonomy, positive relations with others, environmental mastery, purpose in life, and personal growth.[42–44] The items of her Psychological Well-Being Scale are rated using a 6-point scale, ranging from strongly agree to strongly disagree. Samples of these questions are provided in Table 10.6.

Affect Balance Scale

The Affect Balance Scale (ABS) contains 10 yes/no questions. Five questions have a positive affect, and five have a negative affect.[45] The ABS is used as an index of well-being or happiness. It has been successfully used to measure the effects of group treatment and other approaches to aphasia.[46, 47]

Interactive Communication Scales

Lyon uses Interactive Communication Scales for measuring the comfort, confidence, connectedness, and pleasure experienced by persons with aphasia in communicative interactions.[48] These Likert-type scales, shown in Figure 10.3, can be used to measure the psychosocial effects of group treatment with individual patients.

Table 10.6
Sample questions from Psychological Well-Being Scale.

Autonomy	Sometimes I change the way I act or think to be more like those around me.
Environmental mastery	In general, I feel I am in charge of the situation in which I live.
Personal growth	I am not interested in activities that will expand my horizons.
Positive relations with others	Most people see me as loving and affectionate.
Purpose in life	I feel good when I think of what I've done in the past and what I hope to do in the future.
Self-acceptance	When I look at the story of my life, I am pleased with how things have turned out.

Source: Reprinted with permission from CD Ryff. Beyond Ponce de Leon and life satisfaction: new directions in quest of successful aging. Int J Behav Dev 1989;12:35.

Documenting Activity

The handicap of aphasia affects patient and family. Often the patient and his or her significant other stop participating in activities they once enjoyed. If group treatment fosters the resumption of activities such as going to church, eating out, and playing cards with friends, that should be documented. Fox and Fried-Oken ask a family member to complete an Activity Level Assessment similar to that shown in Figure 10.4.[49] This assessment allows the clinician to rate the patient's level of participation in various leisure and other activities on a prestroke and pre- and post-treatment basis.

Satisfaction Surveys

Yerxa and colleagues have developed an instrument, the Satisfaction Performance Scaled Questionnaire, that can be used to assess the activity of individuals with poststroke disability in their environments.[50] Lyon et al. and others have modified Ryff's Psychosocial Well-Being Scales to assess life satisfaction of aphasic stroke patients, communication partners, and family members.[46, 51] The unique features of these modifications allow the scales to be used with patients

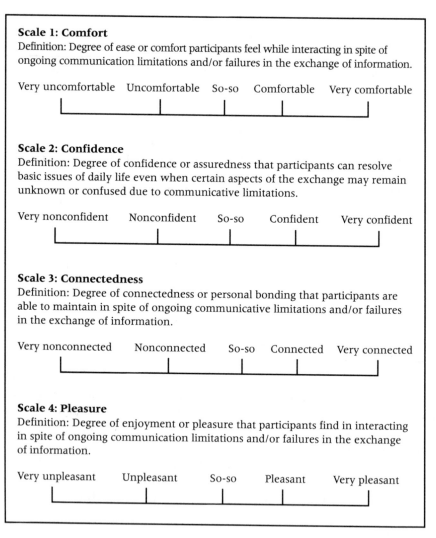

Figure 10.3
Interactive Communication Scales. (Reprinted with permission from J Lyon. Treating Real-Life Functionality in a Couple Coping with Severe Aphasia. In N Helm-Estabrooks, AL Holland [eds], Approaches to the Treatment of Aphasia. San Diego: Singular, 1998;203.)

with language problems such as aphasia. For example, Lyon et al. provide explicit redundant cues to aid a person with aphasia in responding to questions. For example, the cues, "How at ease are you when you are by yourself?" and "when no one else is around," can be used if a patient did not give a complete response to the question, "How comfortable are you being alone?"

Instructions: Using the codes, select the number that best describes the participant's past and present level of social activity. (Codes: 0 = rarely; 1 = yearly;
2 = monthly; 3 = weekly; 4 = daily.)

How frequently does/ did participant:	At present	During adult life
Listen to a radio program?	_____	_____
Follow finances/investments?	_____	_____
Listen to music?	_____	_____
Watch favorite television programs?	_____	_____
Watch a movie?	_____	_____
Spend time at a hobby?	_____	_____
Play a game with family?	_____	_____
Play a game with friends?	_____	_____
Care for a pet?	_____	_____
Visit others at their homes?	_____	_____
Go out to eat?	_____	_____
Have visitors?	_____	_____
Attend a club or group meeting?	_____	_____
Take a class?	_____	_____
Attend church or synagogue?	_____	_____
Vote?	_____	_____
Travel out of town?	_____	_____

Figure 10.4
Oregon Health Science University Activity Level Assessment. (Information from
L Fox and M Fried-Oken, personal communication, 1997.)

The Code-Muller Protocols provide a rapid, simple objective means
of obtaining information from a patient with aphasia regarding his or
her psychosocial adjustment to aphasia.[52] The patient responds to
open-ended questions (e.g., Do you think the ability to work will
. . . ?) in 10 psychosocial areas using a 5-point scale: 0 = get much
worse, 1 = get a little worse, 2 = stay the same, 3 = improve a little,
and 4 = improve a lot. The questionnaire can be administered to the
patient and any significant others in the patient's life. The clinician
can construct profiles that measure features of optimism (e.g., what
will be accomplished in therapy) and congruity. Congruity measure-
ments compare sets of scores from individuals (e.g., patient, significant other, friend).

FINAL COMMENTS ON MONTHLY DOCUMENTATION

The objective measurement of how group treatment improves the communicative and psychosocial functioning of patients with aphasia on a month-to-month basis is the heart of the documentation process. Clinicians have long lamented that documentation takes too much time and that appropriate tools are not available for documenting the subtle and not-so-subtle changes in performances of patients with aphasia that is often chronic. However, many options are available for choosing a documentation strategy that will reflect therapeutic benefits. Few are so time-consuming that they cannot be carried out on a regular basis. Scales, questionnaires, and data-tracking forms are continually being developed by clinicians seeking to improve their documentation practices and to be more objective in what they report. We have only to look at what is available, make a wise decision about what and how to document, and to act decisively.

REFERENCES

1. Marshall RC. Documentation Strategies in Medical Speech Pathology: Seizing the Moment. Paper presented at the American Speech-Language-Hearing Association Convention. Seattle, November 1996.
2. Collins M. Diagnosis and Treatment of Global Aphasia. San Diego: College-Hill, 1986;1.
3. Kertesz A. Western Aphasia Battery. New York: Grune & Stratton, 1982.
4. Porch BE. Porch Index of Communicative Ability. Palo Alto, CA: Consulting Psychologists, 1981.
5. Goodglass H, Kaplan E. The Boston Diagnostic Aphasia Examination. Philadelphia: Lea & Febiger, 1983.
6. Schuell HM. The Minnesota Test for Differential Diagnosis of Aphasia. Minneapolis: University of Minnesota Press, 1972.
7. Lincoln NB, Ells P. A shortened version of the PICA. Br J Disord Commun 1980;15:183.
8. DiSimoni FG, Keith RL, Holt DL, Darley FL. Practicality of shortening the Porch Index of Communicative Ability. J Speech Hear Res 1975;18:478.
9. Schuell HM. A short examination for aphasia. Neurology 1957;7:625.
10. Marshall RC. Problem-focused group treatment for clients with mild aphasia. Am J Speech-Lang Pathol 1993;2:31.
11. Avent J. Group treatment in aphasia using cooperative learning methods. J Med Speech-Lang Pathol 1997;5:9.
12. Avent J. Manual of Cooperative Group Treatment for Aphasia. Boston: Butterworth–Heinemann, 1997;1.

13. Yorkston KM, Beukelman DR. An analysis of connected speech samples of aphasic and normal speakers. J Speech Hear Disord 1980;45:27.
14. Menn L, Ramsburger G, Helm-Estabrooks N. A linguistic measure for aphasic narratives. Aphasiology 1994;8:343.
15. Nicholas LE, Brookshire RH. A system for quantifying the informativeness and efficiency of the connected speech of adults with aphasia. J Speech Hear Res 1993;36:338.
16. Blomert L, Kean ML, Koster C, Schokker J. Amsterdam-Nijmegen Everyday Language Test: construction, reliability, and validity. Aphasiology 1994;8:381.
17. DeRenzi E, Ferrari C. The reporter's test: a sensitive measure to detect expressive disturbances in aphasics. Cortex 1978;14:279.
18. DeRenzi E, Vignolo LA. The token test: a sensitive test to detect receptive disturbances in aphasics. Brain 1962;85:665.
19. McDonald S, Pierce S. The 'dice' game: a new test of pragmatic language skills after closed-head injury. Brain Injury 1995;9:255.
20. Chapman S, Ulatowska H, Branch C, Olness G. Summarization in Mild Aphasia: A Potential Index of Cognitive/Linguistic Ability. Paper presented at the 24th Clinical Aphasiology Conference, Traverse City, Michigan, June 1994.
21. Lyon J. Drawing: its value as a communication aid for adults with aphasia. Aphasiology 1995;9:33.
22. Garrett K, Beukelman DR. Changes in the Interaction Patterns of an Individual with Aphasia Given Three Types of Partner Support. In M Lemme (ed), Clinical Aphasiology. Austin, TX: Pro-Ed, 1995;237.
23. Calculator S, Luchko CD. Evaluating the effectiveness of a communication board training program. J Speech Hear Disord 1983;48:185.
24. Functional Independence Measure. New York: State University of New York at Buffalo Research Foundation, 1993.
25. Holland AL. Communicative Activities in Daily Living. Baltimore: University Park Press, 1980.
26. Lomas J, Pickard L, Bester S, et al. The communicative effectiveness index: development and psychometric evaluation of a functional communication measure for adult aphasia. J Speech Hear Disord 1989;54:113.
27. Fratalli C, Thompson C, Holland A, et al. Functional Assessment of Communication Skills for Adults. Rockville, MD: American Speech-Language-Hearing Association, 1996;1.
28. Sarno MT. The Functional Communication Profile. New York: NYU Medical Center, 1969.
29. Wirz R. Revised Edinburgh Functional Communication Profile. Br J Disord Commun 1990;43:11.
30. Payne J. Communication Profile: A Functional Skills Survey. San Antonio, TX: Communication Skill Builders, 1994;1.
31. Lincoln N. The speech questionnaire: an assessment of functional language ability. Int J Rehabil Med 1984;4:114.
32. Fawcus M, Fawcus R. Information transfer in four cases of articulatory apraxia. Aphasiology 1990;4:207.
33. Yorkston KM, Beukelman DR, Flowers C. Efficiency of Information Exchange Between Aphasic Speakers and Communication Partners. In R Brookshire (ed), Clinical Aphasiology Conference Proceedings. Minneapolis: BRK, 1980;96.

34. Marshall RC, Freed DB, Phillips DS. Communicative efficiency in severe aphasia. Aphasiology 1997;11:373.
35. Linebaugh C, Krizer K, Oden S, Meyers P. Reapportionment of Communicative Burden in Aphasia. A Study of Narrative Interactions. In R Brookshire (ed), Clinical Aphasiology Conference Proceedings. Minneapolis: BRK, 1982;4.
36. Bishop D, Pet R. Psychobehavioral problems other than depression in stroke. Top Stroke Rehabil 1995;2:56.
37. Rau MT, Schultz R. The Psychosocial Context of Stroke-Related Communication Disorders in the Elderly. In HK Ulatowska (ed), Aging and Communication: Seminars in Speech and Language. New York: Thieme, 1988;9:117.
38. Lyon J. Communication use and participation in life for adults with aphasia in natural settings. Am J Speech-Lang Pathol 1992;1:7.
39. Lyon J. Coping with Aphasia. San Diego: Singular, 1998;1.
40. Holland AL, Thompson CK. Outcomes Measurement in Aphasia. In C Fratalli (ed), Measuring Outcomes in Speech-Language Pathology. New York: Thieme, 1998;245.
41. Stern RA, Arruda JE, Hooper CR, et al. Visual analog mood scales to measure internal mood state in neurologically impaired patients: description and initial validity evidence. Aphasiology 1996;10:323.
42. Ryff CD. Beyond Ponce de Leon and life satisfaction: new directions in quest of successful aging. Int J Behav Dev 1989;12:35.
43. Ryff CD. Possible selves in adulthood and old age: a tale of shifting horizons. Psychol Aging 1991;6:286.
44. Ryff CD, Essex MJ. Psychological well-being in adulthood and old age: descriptive markers and explanatory processes. Annu Rev Gerontol Geriatr 1991; 11:145.
45. Bradburn N. The Structure of Psychological Well-Being. Chicago: Aldine, 1969;1.
46. Lyon J. Cariski D, Keisler J, et al. Communication partners: enhancing participation in life and communication for adults with aphasia. Aphasiology 1997;11:693.
47. Elman R, Burnstein-Ellis E. Effectiveness of Group Communication Treatment for Individuals with Chronic Aphasia. Paper presented at the American Speech-Language-Hearing Association Convention, Seattle, November 1996.
48. Lyon J. Treating Real-Life Functionality in a Couple Coping with Severe Aphasia. In N Helm-Estabrooks, AL Holland (eds), Approaches to the Treatment of Aphasia. San Diego: Singular, 1998:203.
49. Fox LE, Fried-Oken M. Interactive Group Treatment for Aphasia: An AAC Alternative. Paper presented at Isaac: 7th Biennial Conference of the International Society for Augmentative and Alternative Communication, 1996;390.
50. Yerxa EJ, Burnett-Bealieu SE, Stocking S, Azen S. Development of the satisfaction with performance scaled questionnaire (SPSQ). Am J Occup Ther 1988;42:215.
51. Hoen B, Thelander M, Worsley J. Improvement in psychological well-being of people with aphasia and their families: evaluation of a community-based program. Aphasiology 1997;11:681.
52. Code C, Muller D. Code-Muller Protocols. Kibworth, UK: Far Communications, 1992;1.

11

Social Validation

Social validation is another means of evaluating the clinical significance of changes resulting from a treatment program. In this evaluation, socially relevant behaviors of persons in treatment are compared with that of their peers, and subjective evaluations of the behaviors of interest are obtained from individuals in the patient's natural environment.[1] Social validation is the most recent addition to the clinician's arsenal of documentation weapons. It is, however, an important adjunct to objective measures presented earlier.

OBSERVATION

How can the clinician determine how patients with aphasia communicate in the natural environment if his or her observations are limited to the treatment room? Some field observation is necessary, and we might be surprised by the patient's performance. Some patients perform admirably in the treatment session with support from the clinician, only to suffer breakdowns or fail to communicate in naturalistic situations. Others are remarkably adept at making their needs known in a naturalistic setting, but fare less well on task-specific behaviors of treatment and standardized tests. For example, Simmons et al. found that patients with severe aphasia used certain compensatory strategies in the therapy room, but used these same strategies selectively in naturalistic situations with different communicative partners.[2] Field observation is important in knowing about any discrepancies in a patient's performance in the clinic and naturalistic environments.

Holland, a strong advocate of observation, suggests that observation is a qualitatively helpful method for knowing an aphasic patient better.[3] Seeing the patient with aphasia communicating in situations outside the clinic (e.g., the home, a store, or on the telephone) with different partners (e.g., the spouse, a friend, or a child), and in more

---

Phrases

Check the terms that best describe the aphasic patient's role in the conversation you observed.

1. Participation: Patient was primarily
Active _____   Passive _____

2. Sending and receiving messages: Patient was primarily
A sender _____   A receiver _____   About equal _____

3. Use of questions: Patient was primarily
An answerer _____   An asker _____   About equal _____

4. Leadership: In the conversation with the partner, the patient was primarily
The leader _____   Was led _____   About equal _____

5. Turn taking: In the conversation with the partner, the patient was primarily
Dominant _____   Submissive _____   About equal participation _____

6. Other: Was the person with aphasia primarily
Talking _____   Talked to _____

7. In this conversation, I observed the aphasic person to be
A poor communicator _____   A good communicator _____

Figure 11.1
Descriptive checklist of terms for use in observing functional communication of aphasic persons in conversations. (Data from AL Holland. Observing functional communication of aphasic adults. J Speech Hear Disord 1982;47:50.)

stressful environments (e.g., in a noisy cafeteria or under time pressure), will aid the clinician in setting treatment goals that meet the patient's functional needs.

Holland provides a comprehensive scheme for observing functional communication of adults with aphasia encompassing conversation, comprehension, word-finding, topic initiation, and topic changing skills. The observer (1) selects phrases, similar to those shown in Figure 11.1, to describe an aphasic patient's role in a conversation. (2) The observer rates adequacy of the patient's overall communication in the

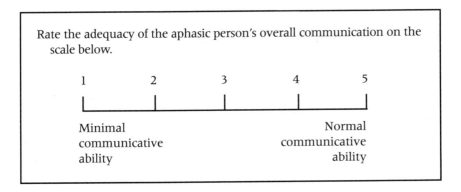

Rate the adequacy of the aphasic person's overall communication on the scale below.

1   2   3   4   5

Minimal   Normal
communicative   communicative
ability   ability

Figure 11.2
Rating scale of overall communication adequacy. (Data from RC Marshall, DB Freed, DS Phillips. Communicative efficiency in severe aphasia. Aphasiology 1997;11:373.)

conversation on a 5-point scale (Figure 11.2). The scale can be used to rate the patient's conversational performance in different situations, with different partners. The clinician may find that rank ordering performances across settings, partners, and so on is helpful. This information could be useful in treatment planning and developing outside assignments for the patient.

In many cases, going to the patient's home for direct observation is not possible. However, ways to study conversational interactions of an aphasic patient communicating in familiar surroundings, such as the home, are available. A unique approach developed by Orange and colleagues examines the conversational repairs in patients with Alzheimer's disease.[4] Patients and their significant others were supplied with videocameras and instructed to record naturally occurring conversational interactions at their discretion in their homes. Most aphasic patients are older. Given the propensity of older persons to buy videocameras to record life events, the clinician may be able to tap this resource or find that some individuals have already recorded communicative interactions in more naturalistic settings.

USE OF NAIVE RATERS AND PEER GROUPS

Some clinicians obtain informal social validation information by soliciting family members' opinions about how a patient is communicating at home. Talking to family members is another means of determining whether a patient is better off than he or she was before group treatment. A greater degree of objectivity can be obtained by developing a rating procedure for the adequacy of specific target behaviors or by actually instructing the family member or other rater how to rate functional performance with scales such as the Communicative Effectiveness Index (CETI),[5] American Speech-Language-Hearing Association Functional Assessment of Communication Skills for Adults (ASHA-FACS),[6] and others discussed in Chapter 10. Outside, unbiased evaluators of a given task behavior can also be taught to evaluate specific target behaviors. For example, Doyle et al. trained naive listeners to make judgments of adequacy on taped speech samples of patients with Broca's aphasia.[7] An adequate response was defined as "one that communicated an unambiguous message that was appropriate to the context (i.e., the experimenter's question and a corresponding picture)." Another study by Marshall et al. trained naive judges to make ratings of communicative efficiency and degree of communicative burden assumed by the partner in message exchange tasks involving severely aphasic subjects (see Figure 11.2).[8]

Peer-group comparison methods can also be useful in assessing the social validity of use of social conversation (e.g., greetings, introductions), doing specific tasks (e.g., writing a check), and communicating in real-life interaction situations (e.g., ordering food at a restaurant). Naive raters would be asked to compare the aphasic person's performance with those of normal adults. Thompson and Byrne have demonstrated how a peer-group comparison method can be used to assess the social validity in the use of social conversations of adults with aphasia.[9]

SOCIAL VALIDATION QUESTIONNAIRES

The clinician seeking to socially validate the benefits of treatment might consider developing a questionnaire for this purpose. Table 11.1 reflects a sample of questions to collect social validation data during treatment.[10] Table 11.2 exhibits a questionnaire that would provide social validation information as a patient exits treatment.[11] The latter might also be seen as a measure of patient or customer satisfaction. Useful also in this vein is a one-page ASHA questionnaire designed to measure customer satisfaction.[12]

CLIENT SELF-REPORTS

Client self-reports are also useful measures of social validation. Marshall asks persons unfamiliar with the patient (e.g., first-year graduate stu-

Table 11.1
Sample of questions used to elicit social validation data during treatment.

Did you do anything new or fun since we last met?
Have you faced any recent challenges in your life?
Have there been any changes in your activities?
How is this therapy helping you away from the clinic?
Have you felt different about your communication skills in any speaking situation lately?

Source: Reprinted with permission from S Klingman. Cooperative Group Treatment for Individuals with Mild Aphasia. In J Avent (ed), Manual of Cooperative Group Treatment for Aphasia. Boston: Butterworth–Heinemann, 1997;19.

Table 11.2
Social validation questionnaire administered at completion of therapy.

---

1. Do you feel that you have made improvements by participating in this treatment?
2. If you feel that you made improvements, do you feel that it was worth the time and effort you put into it?
3. Did you enjoy this therapy?
4. Would you recommend it to someone else who has similar language difficulties?
5. What was the worst part of this experience?
6. What was the best part of this experience?
7. Do you think working with a partner was helpful? If so, how do you think it helped?
8. Were there any disadvantages to working with a therapy partner?
9. Has this therapy had any impact on your communication or life outside the clinic?
10. Do you have any suggestions to improve this therapy approach?

Source: Reprinted with permission from P Hatch. Advanced Cooperative Group Treatment for Individuals with Mild Aphasia. In J Avent (ed), Manual of Cooperative Group Treatment for Aphasia. Boston: Butterworth–Heinemann, 1997;95.

dents) to conduct an unstructured interview with the patient.[13, 14] The objectives of the interview are to determine how the patient communicates in daily life. Interview information from year to year is compared. Patients frequently report doing things in one year that were impossible the prior year. For example, one patient reported resuming weekly poker games with friends. This type of information is in keeping with Lyon's view of "the journey of aphasia" as one that lasts for years.[15]

A more formal measure of social validation that falls into the self-report group is the Problem Solving Inventory (PSI).[16] This set of scales provides an estimate of a patient's ability to solve real-life problems. The PSI is useful in assessing an individual's perceptions of his or her problem-solving behaviors and attitudes. It contains 35 items and three scales: problem solving and confidence, approach-avoidance style, and personal control. A total PSI score is used as a general index of problem-solving ability.

An informal social validation measure to assess problem solving of brain-injured subjects with aphasia used by Marshall et al. appears in Figure 11.3.[17] This scale is similar to that used with the CETI. The patient's significant other is asked to rate the patient's problem-solving abilities using this scale.

INTAKE AND EXIT INTERVIEWS

Pictures are worth a thousand words. Clinicians seeking to socially validate the effects of treatment may find videotaping a brief intake interview with the patient before starting group treatment to be helpful. Subsequent brief interviews using questions similar to those shown in Table 11.2 can be conducted during treatment and when treatment ends.[12] This information is also useful from the standpoint of social validation. It may be helpful when explaining to the administrative powers of the health care organization exactly how speech-language services help your patients.

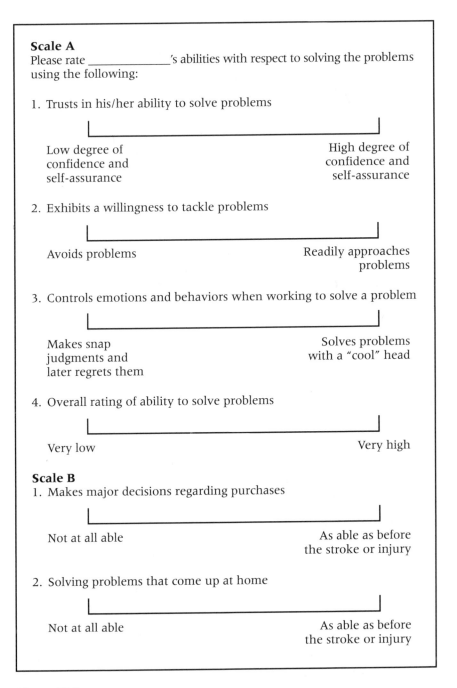

Scale A
Please rate _____'s abilities with respect to solving the problems using the following:

1. Trusts in his/her ability to solve problems

Low degree of confidence and self-assurance   High degree of confidence and self-assurance

2. Exhibits a willingness to tackle problems

Avoids problems   Readily approaches problems

3. Controls emotions and behaviors when working to solve a problem

Makes snap judgments and later regrets them   Solves problems with a "cool" head

4. Overall rating of ability to solve problems

Very low   Very high

Scale B
1. Makes major decisions regarding purchases

Not at all able   As able as before the stroke or injury

2. Solving problems that come up at home

Not at all able   As able as before the stroke or injury

Figure 11.3
Rating scales for use by significant others to rate problem-solving ability. Note lines should be 100 mm in length. (Data from RC Marshall, C Morelli, K King-Iden, C Karow. Question-Asking Strategies of TBI and Non–Brain-Damaged Subjects. Paper presented at the Clinical Aphasiology Conference, Ashville, NC, June 1998.)

3. Weighing all alternatives before making decisions

Not at all able   As able as before
                                         the stroke or injury

4. Developing and carrying out a plan for solving a problem that comes up at home

Not at all able   As able as before
                                         the stroke or injury

5. Altering a plan when something goes wrong

Not at all able   As able as before
                                         the stroke or injury

Figure 11.3 (continued)

REFERENCES

1. Brookshire R. Introduction to Neurogenic Communication Disorders (5th ed). St. Louis: Mosby, 1997.
2. Simmons-Mackie NN, Damico JS. Reformulating the definition of compensatory strategies in aphasia. Aphasiology 1997;11:761.
3. Holland AL. Observing functional communication of aphasia adults. J Speech Hear Disord 1982;47:50.
4. Orange JB, Lubinski R, Higgenbotham DJ. Conversational repair by individuals with dementia of the Alzheimer's type. J Speech Hear Res 1996;39:881.
5. Lomas J, Pickard L, Bester S, et al. The communicative effectiveness index: development and psychometric evaluation of a functional communication measure for adult aphasia. J Speech Hear Disord 1989;54:113.
6. Fratalli C, Thompson C, Holland A, et al. Functional Assessment of Communication Skills for Adults. Rockville, MD: American Speech-Language-Hearing Association, 1996.
7. Doyle PJ, Goldstein H, Bourgeois MS. Experimental analysis of syntax training in Broca's aphasia: a generalization and social validation study. J Speech Hear Res 1987;52:143.
8. Marshall RC, Freed DB, Phillips DS. Communicative efficiency in severe aphasia. Aphasiology 1997;11:373.
9. Thompson C, Byrne M. Across Setting Generalization of Social Conventions in Aphasia. In R Brookshire (ed), Clinical Aphasiology Conference Proceedings. Minneapolis: BRK, 1984;132.

10. Klingman S. Cooperative Group Treatment for Individuals with Mild Aphasia. In J Avent (ed), Manual of Cooperative Group Treatment for Aphasia. Boston: Butterworth–Heinemann, 1997;19.

11. Hatch P. Advanced Cooperative Group Treatment for Individuals with Mild Aphasia. In J Avent (ed), Manual of Cooperative Group Treatment for Aphasia. Boston: Butterworth–Heinemann, 1997;95.

12. American Speech-Language-Hearing Association. Functional Communication Measures. Rockville, MD: American Speech-Language-Hearing Association, 1987.

13. Marshall RC. Problem-focused group treatment for clients with mild aphasia. Am J Speech-Lang Pathol 1993;2:31.

14. Marshall RC. A Problem-Focused Group Treatment Program for Clients with Mild Aphasia. In R Elman (ed), Group Treatment for Aphasia: The Expert Clinician's Approach. Boston: Butterworth–Heinemann, 1999.

15. Lyon J. Coping with Aphasia. San Diego: Singular, 1997.

16. Heppner PP. The Problem Solving Inventory. Palo Alto, CA: Consulting Psychologists 1988.

17. Marshall, RC, Morelli C, King-Iden K, Karow C. Question-Asking Strategies of TBI and Non–Brain-Damaged Subjects. Paper presented at the Clinical Aphasiology Conference, Ashville, NC, June 1998.

12

Some Final Comments

Those involved in aphasia group treatment programs have "the passion." A noninclusive list of persons who appear committed to the group treatment process includes Jon Lyon, Roberta Elman, Ellen Burnstein-Ellis, Audrey Holland, Pagie Beeson, Jackie Hinckley, Mary Beth Clark, Lynn Fox, Kathy Garrett, Tom Hintgen, Jan Avent, and Robert Marshall in this country; Aura Kagan, Lillian Gailey, and Guylaine LeDorze in Canada; and Maria Pachalska, Peter Wahrborg, Carol Pound, Susie Parr, and Sally Byng in Europe. One develops the passion by seeing how aphasic people respond to group treatment and how their lives are positively affected by it.

Getting caught up in the emotions associated with aphasic persons' positive response to group treatment is easy. For example, Deanie Vogel (personal communication, 1998), a speech-language pathologist who provided treatment to many of the aphasic patients who were subjects in the Veterans Administration Cooperative Study found that one of the favorite activities of the group was watching movies of horse races in which the patients placed a bet and expressed their rationale for their choice of horses. Anyone who has seen his or her share of aphasic patients knows that this activity is probably much more interesting, exciting, and meaningful to the patient than pointing to one of six common objects in a field of 10 with 80% accuracy. Becoming passionate about group treatment is not difficult.

The passion and dedication of those involved in group treatment of aphasia is evident in the publication of new textbooks.[1, 2] This book can be included in this category. Increasing space is now given to group treatment in general textbooks on neurogenic communication disorders and aphasia.[3–6] Presentations on group treatment are becoming more abundant at national and international professional meetings such as the American Speech-Language-Hearing Association and Clinical Aphasiology conferences.

Most group therapy "junkies" like myself understand that the renewed interest in this activity is driven by financial constraints on health care imposed by managed care. Perhaps we are thinking that this is our moment—that it is time to go for it. I must be completely candid. I wrote this book because I believe that more patients with aphasia will be seen in groups in the near future and hope that clinicians who see these patients will read this book and use it to provide the highest quality of group treatment services.

FEARS FOR THE FUTURE

Along with the emotions associated with the renewed interest in aphasia group treatment and what appears to be a desire to have more groups, arise some fears for the future. We should remember the old adage: Be careful what you wish for. In this instance, what is being wished for is the opportunity to treat more patients with aphasia in group situations. Remember that group treatment is not a panacea. It is a viable treatment approach for some, but not all, aphasic patients.

Abuses

When medical speech-pathology programs began to truly thrive in the early 1970s, Joseph Wepman sounded a warning: He cautioned that clinicians would need to do battle with health care and hospital administrators over the when and how of aphasia treatment.[7] Wepman's prediction appears to have come true. Today's aphasia clinicians need to balance what is best for the patient with what is best for the company. Thus, they are challenged to advocate for services to patients with aphasia and to guard against the use of management practices based on factors other than quality of patient care.

In Chapter 4, the cost of providing group treatment was approached very rationally. Health care organizations, however, are businesses. Businesses are concerned with profits. Group treatment, however, should not simply be a way to increase the bottom line. Chapter 4 shows that enormous profits are realized if aphasic patients are seen in groups and charged at individual rates. To do this would be abuse, plain and simple. No patient in group treatment receives the amount of attention that is possible in individual treatment. Charges for group treatment can be fair and equitable to payer and patient and still permit the organization to profit.

Expected cutbacks in medical care dollars could mean fewer jobs and perhaps lower pay for speech-language pathologists. Some clinicians are concerned that clinicians who do have jobs will be asked to treat more patients. This do-more-with-less philosophy is dangerous. If an organization seeks to compensate for its human resources cutbacks by putting all patients in groups because no one is available to see them individually, that would constitute a form of abuse.

Group treatment should not be used in lieu of individual treatment; rather it is a viable alternative. If group treatment can accomplish the same results at a lower cost than individual treatment, it should be the method of choice. A group session, however, is not the place to assess a patient's deficits, to identify strengths and weaknesses, or to set treatment goals. For problems as complex as aphasia, a certain amount of individual assessment is necessary to decide whether group treatment is an appropriate and more cost-effective alternative. Abandoning individual treatment in favor of group treatment is just as abusive as seeing all patients individually. Patient needs should dictate the course of action.

On the positive side, there are indeed indications the health care organizations and those who provide aphasia treatment services can work together as partners for the betterment of the lives of aphasic persons and their families. This is clearly apparent in the successes of the community aphasia groups in this country and abroad and the fact that funding has been obtained to support these programs.[8–10]

Group Treatment as a Microcosm of Individual Treatment

Traditional individual aphasia treatment involves language stimulation and working on specific tasks (e.g., word-picture matching, naming, sentence completion, or repetition). Although functionally based therapies now seem more popular, much of what is undertaken with a person with aphasia is still based on tenets of the stimulation approach.[11] Another of my concerns for the future is that group treatment will become a place where individuals perform matching, naming, and other tasks that have dominated aphasia treatment approaches for decades. A paper by Eales and Pring suggests that this idea is not unrealistic.[12] If these activities become the focus of group treatment, it is quite possible that speech-language pathology assistants (SLP-As) will be assigned these group functions. This change should be unacceptable to those responsible for the management of persons with aphasia. Aphasic patients who are still able to profit from stimulation approaches need individualized, carefully planned programs. Moreover, a significant amount of experience, training, and clinical acumen is required to facilitate a group. No report of group treatment speaks of paraprofessionals such as SLP-As running groups. In fact, many group programs use a combination of professionals in providing group treatment.

HOPES

When one is passionate about something, he or she thinks about what is possible. These thoughts constitute vision, hopes, and even dreams about the future. Lyon's view of the patient and the significant other setting out on a journey after a stroke that causes aphasia sets the stage to address some hopes.[13] He divides this journey into phases: hospitalization, rehabilitation, dismissal from formal treatment, 1 year postonset, and 2 years postonset. Others see the journey as lasting even longer.[14] Ignoring the issue of the length of the journey, most clinicians would agree with Lyon on this point. The journey that the aphasic person and caregiver take has several rest stops, side trips, and detours that are a part of the poststroke improvement process. A second point made by Lyon—that the aphasic person will improve so long as he or she keeps working at it—warrants serious contemplation. Groups provide a place to do this work.

Research

Aphasia treatment will always be under scrutiny with respect to what its benefits are for patients. Group treatment will not be exempted from this scrutiny. To do so would be a serious abrogation of professional responsibility. A number of writers have pointed out the need to conduct outcome studies of group treatment programs and methods.[15–17] This research is well under way.

Training

Aphasia treatment has a long history of being deficit-specific. Deficit-specific assessment and treatment methods continue to be what most university professors teach their students to do with persons with aphasia. It is becoming very apparent that these types of treatments are not having a significant effect on the aphasic patient's day-to-day communications and that what we thought might be an appropriate compensatory strategy for the patient in the clinic sometimes has little value in the outside world. The central problem becomes one of teaching students how to make the shift from impairment-based treatment to helping aphasic people live better. Again, there is growing evidence that present-day aphasiologists are taking this need seriously.

Psychosocial Issues

We know that aphasia wreaks havoc with many areas of psychosocial functioning; this disorder erodes the patient's sense of self.[18] Several excellent resources exist that clearly document the psychosocial consequences of aphasia.[19–22] Although an in-depth discussion of the psychosocial consequences of aphasia is beyond the scope of this book, if these consequences are reduced by group treatment, we need to know why and how. For example, clinicians should determine how persons with aphasia improve after resuming former activities. Some writers have provided guidelines for studying psychosocial problems in aphasia, but we have a long way to go in developing measures that reflect the psychosocial benefits of group work with aphasic patients.[23, 24] Let us hope this work is done soon.

A GROUP FOR EVERY PATIENT

A little dreaming never hurts anyone. Visualize a world where every patient with aphasia who wants to be involved in a group has that opportunity. Let your imagination go, and visualize this opportunity being available for as long as the aphasia exists—for life. Group treatment may be possible without raising taxes, converting to a socialized medical care system, or resorting to any other drastic actions.

Think about basing group treatment on a level-of-care system. Level one would represent for the patient a viable alternative to individual treatment. Here, the patient would be expected to improve on communication and behavioral indices at a rate equivalent to individual treatment. This service would be fully funded.

Level two group treatment would address what Simmons-Mackie called the *discharge dilemma of aphasia treatment*.[25] These patients have no funds to pay for continued individual therapy or are no longer making sufficient progress in individual therapy to justify its cost. Nevertheless, these patients are capable of making further gains, and they warrant professional attention. The group provides treatment at a lower cost and for a longer period than would be the case if the patient were seen individually. The clinician remains obligated to measure the effects of treatment, but not as often or with the expectations of improvement over time as with level one patients.

Level three would provide ongoing support, guidance, opportunities, and education for aphasic persons and their families over the life span. Aphasia is a long-term problem. These services help the patient maintain any gains. They provide hope. Community agencies, recovered stroke victims, stroke clubs, and organizations such as the National Aphasia Association recognize this long-term need. Professionals, particularly those proficient in the treatment of aphasia, should become involved in these endeavors. According to present health care policies, these services are not reimbursable. Perhaps we could find a way. I doubt that you could find an aphasic person or a member of his or her family that would say this continued service does not help.

FINAL IMAGES

I would like to end by suggesting that clinical aphasiologists become committed to group treatment for aphasia rather than just involved in the process. An explanation is warranted here. A top-flight tennis professional who had just won a major championship was being interviewed by a sportswriter. The player was asked, "What do you feel is responsible for the great improvements in your play over the last 2 years?" The player answered, "I used to be involved in tennis. Now I'm committed to it." The sportswriter said, "Please explain." The tennis player answered, "It's like bacon and eggs for breakfast. The chicken is involved, but the pig is committed."

REFERENCES

1. Elman R. Group Treatment for Aphasia. The Expert Clinician's Approach. Boston: Butterworth–Heinemann, 1999.
2. Avent J. Manual of Cooperative Group Treatment for Aphasia. Boston: Butterworth–Heinemann, 1997.
3. Holland AL, Forbes M. Aphasia Treatment: World Perspectives. London: Chapman & Hall, 1993.
4. Brookshire R. An Introduction to Neurogenic Communication Disorders (5th ed). St. Louis: Mosby, 1997.
5. Chapey R. Language Intervention Strategies in Adult Aphasia (3rd ed). Baltimore: Williams & Wilkins, 1994.
6. Wallace GJ. Adult Aphasia Rehabilitation. Boston: Butterworth–Heinemann, 1996.
7. Wepman JM. Aphasia therapy: a new look. J Speech Hear Disord 1972;37:303.

8. Kagan A. Revealing the competence of aphasic adults through conversation. A challenge of health care professionals. Topics Stroke Rehab 1995;2:1.

9. Hintgen T, Clark MB, Radichel T. Development of a community-based aphasia program. Poster session at the Clinical Aphasiology Conference, Asheville, NC, June 1998.

10. Pound C. Power, partnerships, and practicalities: developing cost-effective support services for living with aphasia. Paper presented at the Clinical Aphasiology Conference, Asheville, NC, June 1998.

11. Duffy J. Schuell's Stimulation Approach to Rehabilitation. In R Chapey (ed), Language Intervention Strategies in Adult Aphasia (3rd ed). Baltimore: Williams & Wilkins, 1994;146.

12. Eales C, Pring T. Using individual and group therapy to remediate word finding difficulties. Aphasiology (in press).

13. Lyon J. Coping with Aphasia. San Diego: Singular, 1998.

14. Marshall RC. Problem-Focused Groups for Clients with Mild Aphasia. In R Elman (ed), Group Treatment for Aphasia. The Expert Clinician's Approach. Boston: Butterworth–Heinemann, 1999.

15. Kearns K. Group Therapy for Aphasia: Theoretical and Practical Considerations. In R Chapey (ed), Language Intervention Strategies in Adult Aphasia (3rd ed). Baltimore: Williams & Wilkins, 1994;304.

16. Fawcus M. Group Therapy: A Learning Situation. In C Code, D Muller (eds), Aphasia Therapy. London: Arnold, 1983;113.

17. Aten J. Group therapy for aphasic patients: let's show that it works. Aphasiology 1991;5:559.

18. Brumfitt S. Losing your sense of self: what aphasia can do. Aphasiology 1993;7:569.

19. LeDorze G, Brassard C. A description of the consequences of aphasia on aphasic persons and their relatives and friends based on the WHO model of chronic diseases. Aphasiology 1995;9:239.

20. Sarno MT. Aphasia rehabilitation: psychosocial and ethical considerations. Aphasiology 7;4:321.

21. Sarno MT. Quality of life in the first post-stroke year. Aphasiology 1997;11:665.

22. Rau MT, Schultz R. The Psychosocial Context of Stroke-Related Communication Disorders in the Elderly. In H Ulatowska (ed), Aging and Communication Seminars in Speech and Language. New York: Thieme, 1988;9:117.

23. Herrman M. Studying psychosocial problems in aphasia: some conceptual and methodological considerations. Aphasiology 1997;11:717.

24. Wahrborg P. Assessment and Management of Emotional and Psychosocial Reactions to Brain Damage and Aphasia. San Diego: Singular, 1991.

25. Simmons-Mackie NN, Damico JS. Reformulating the definition of compensatory strategies in aphasia. Aphasiology 1997;11:761.

Index

Note: Page numbers followed by *t* indicate tables; page numbers followed by *f* indicate figures.